Remembering Home

Remembering Home

Rediscovering the Self in Dementia

HABIB CHAUDHURY

The Johns Hopkins University Press
Baltimore

© 2008 The Johns Hopkins University Press
All rights reserved. Published 2008
Printed in the United States of America on acid-free paper
2   4   6   8   9   7   5   3   1

The Johns Hopkins University Press
2715 North Charles Street
Baltimore, Maryland 21218-4363
www.press.jhu.edu

All illustrations used with permission

Library of Congress Cataloging-in-Publication Data
Chaudhury, Habib.
Remembering home : rediscovering the self in dementia /
Habib Chaudhury.
p. ; cm.
Includes bibliographical references and index.
ISBN-13: 978-0-8018-8826-7 (hardcover : alk. paper)
ISBN-13: 978-0-8018-8827-4 (pbk. : alk. paper)
ISBN-10: 0-8018-8826-3 (hardcover : alk. paper)
ISBN-10: 0-8018-8827-1 (pbk. : alk. paper)
1. Dementia—Patients—Care—Psychological aspects. 2. Dementia—
Patients—Long term care—Psychological aspects. 3. Home—
Psychological aspects. 4. Reminiscing in old age. 5. Identity
(Psychology) in old age. 6. Self. 1. Title.
[DNLM: 1. Dementia—therapy. 2. Dementia—psychology.
3. Homes for the Aged. 4. Social Environment. WM 220 C496r 2008]
RC521.C479 2008
362.196'8—dc22   2007040153

A catalog record for this book is available from the British Library.

Special discounts are available for bulk purchases of this book.
For more information, please contact Special Sales at 410-516-6936 or
specialsales@press.jhu.edu.

The Johns Hopkins University Press uses environmentally friendly
book materials, including recycled text paper that is composed of
at least 30 percent post-consumer waste, whenever possible.
All of our book papers are acid-free, and our jackets and
covers are printed on paper with recycled content.

CONTENTS

This book discusses the importance of memories of home in the lives of persons with dementia. It provides a glimpse of the richness and variety of life experiences that are associated with homes, it proposes home as a topic and theme for relating to persons with dementia, and it offers practical suggestions for conducting small-group sessions with persons who have dementia using their own home experiences as triggers for recollection. This book's primary audience is health care professionals and activity leaders in long-term care facilities, assisted living facilities, and adult day centers. Academics, family members, and anyone interested in understanding and relating to the person behind the dementia may find the book useful.

To make a case for the significance of memories of home in persons with dementia and for the potential of reconnecting with the self, one must understand and appreciate the essence and human foundation of the person with dementia. As the person faces challenges in communication and behavior, it is not uncommon for those around that person to treat, interact with, and think of him or her as less than a person. The first two chapters of the book discuss reconsidering the person in dementia, fundamentally valuing a transcendent self beyond expressed memories and socially accepted behavioral patterns, and viewing the possibility of home as a theme for reaching out to that self. The third chapter presents themes in the recollection of homes and related life experiences expressed by family members of residents with dementia in care facilities. Home biographies of the residents and themes emerging from guided conversations with residents form chapter 4. The final chapter provides strategies and suggestions for caregivers to develop home stories and conduct guided conversation sessions with persons who have dementia.

The book grounds practical suggestions for caregivers and staff members in the understanding that there are places, especially homes, in many of our lives that provide a cognitive and emotional foundation of our life experiences. If we recognize the importance of life histories for people with dementia, home is a useful theme in beginning that journey of recognition, understanding, and caring. There is much about the inner world of dementia that we do not know; one approach to learning more is to explore pathways that might lead to that inner world. This is an attempt to provide some directions on the pathway of home to the self.

I would like express my sincere gratitude to the residents, family members, and staff who took part in the empirical portion of this study. Special thanks to those families who inspired me with their enthusiasm and support for this project.

Various portions of this work were supported by multiple organizations or groups. Initial work was supported by the Institute on Aging and Environment at the University of Wisconsin–Milwaukee. The supportive environment of that institute was essential for the launching of this study. I am deeply indebted to the Centre for Research on Personhood in Dementia at the University of British Columbia for its multifaceted support. Thanks to Simon Fraser University (SFU) / Social Science Humanities Research Council Small Grant program and SFU Publications Funds for making the study feasible at the latter stages. Finally, I would like to extend my thanks to the anonymous reviewers for their invaluable feedback.

Remembering Home

CHAPTER ONE

Self and Dementia

Reframing the Relational Landscape

I sit at my worktable, a still world around me, and stare
at the wall, empty of decoration. I become lost in the
vocabulary of silence. Thoughts squiggle and writhe into
sentences that disappear before they can be acknowledged.
—*Thomas DeBaggio*, Losing My Mind *(2002)*

The concept and reality of "self" is a debated area in various humanities and social science disciplines. Perhaps it is most contested and am-
biguous in the context of persons living with dementia. When much of
memory is not apparent, communication skills are impaired, personality
has changed, and behaviors are challenging, is the "person" who was
there before dementia still there? Even though the person does not communicate in the same way as before, is he or she still there but beyond
reach? Or has the person we've known transformed into a different person altogether?

There is evidence that many persons with dementia respond positively
to various activities, such as therapeutic (e.g., music and art), vocational
(e.g., household or professional activities), and reminiscence (e.g., verbal
or art-based) (e.g., Harris, 2002). With occasional flashes—a smile, a look
of recognition, a moment of lucidity, a gesture—the person hidden behind
the condition of dementia comes through, reminding us that he or she is
still there but struggling with communication, anxiety, and frustration.

In the last decade or so, several perspectives have articulated the impact of social relations on the behaviors of persons with dementia. Most

notably, the well-known psychologist Tom Kitwood, in his groundbreaking book *Dementia Reconsidered: The Person Comes First,* articulated the notion of malignant social psychology, describing vividly how our interactions with the person who has dementia are significant in creating the experience of dementia. Several other publications have pointed out the existence of the self behind dementia and the social process in which the self is undermined (e.g., Hughes et al., 2006; Sabat, 2002, 2001). It is critical that we evaluate the quality of relationships and interactions between care providers and persons with dementia and identify the negative ways in which the person with dementia is treated and responded to without (or with) the conscious knowledge of the caregiver. The personal detractors and enhancers such as those identified in Dementia Care Mapping (from Bradford Dementia Group) are one of the ways in which we can begin to understand the quality of life for a person with dementia living in a care facility; with conviction and will, this understanding can be translated into responsive care practices and interactions.

It is important to recognize that this positive person-centered work is difficult given the reality of the high workload of care aides and nursing and activity staff members. An organizational culture change in dementia care is needed to develop a place where the person with dementia is valued and responded to with respect, dignity, and compassion. The culture of care that supports care practices focusing on the person's remaining abilities needs to be constantly guided by the recognition of the understanding and appreciation of the self who is still there behind the veil of the condition of dementia. The self that exists must be acknowledged, appreciated, and responded to at multiple levels.

We can conceptualize the self as a nested phenomenon with multiple layers. At the outer level are the physical body and the sensory experiences. At the next level we can refer to the representation of self as self-identity as the aggregate of personal memories and social personas. Beyond the cognitive and memory structure of self-identity is the part of the self that is largely ineffable: the spiritual identity or the soul. And the individual soul can be thought of as being sustained by the spirit that transcends the individual soul. This latter aspect of self is in recognition of the intangible essence of *being*. It is critical to bring this *essence of humanness* as the ontological foundation into our understanding of the self in dementia. Recognition, understanding, and appreciation of the self that is behind the "difficult" behaviors, frustrations, anxieties, and loss of memory can provide us the platform on which to build and maintain relationships with persons who have dementia.

As much as we appreciate and work with the remaining capacities of the person within the condition of dementia, there are times for caregivers—family members, friends, or health care professionals—when it is easy to become overwhelmed by the stress and challenges of caregiving. At those times in particular, the belief in and understanding of the reality of a self that transcends memory, social context, and behaviors can help us refocus our attention onto what it really means to be human. Kitwood's notion of transcendence of self, articulated in *Dementia Reconsidered* (1997), offers a key foundational framework for re-recognizing the person who underlies the behavioral challenges in dementia. Although Kitwood distanced his premise of personhood or self from that of the religious traditions, perhaps to reach wider audience, it is useful to reconnect with the spiritual perspectives that affirm the transcendency and universality of the self.

This self can be likened to the *Atman* in Vedic tradition, the *Ruh* in Sufism, or the *Ein Sof* in the tradition of Kabbalah in terms of a *being* that has qualities beyond the individual we know. Our perceptions of, attitudes to, and behaviors toward others are largely shaped by the *premise* of the relationship. For example, a family member's quality of interaction with the loved one with dementia is guided by the nature and characteristics of the relationship between the two individuals. Similarly, the quality of care provided to a person with dementia in a care facility is shaped by, among other factors, the premise that defines that relationship. In this latter context, the premise is influenced by staff members' training, organizational policies, staff members' personal traits, and so on. In both these examples, an apparently simple yet powerful shift in the caregiver's perspective on the identity of the person with dementia can have a strong impact on the caregiver's attitude, values, and actions. This shift concerns the basis of the person's identity or self: an understanding of the person's identity that is firmly rooted in a place that not only affirms the person's remaining memories and life experiences, as well as the challenges that have been brought on by the condition of dementia, but also goes beyond and identifies the spiritual basis of the person's self-identity. To honor life, affirm life, and transcend the sufferings of life, one needs to reconnect, both intellectually and emotionally, with the sacredness of life. In this process of honoring and affirming the sacred self that is behind the condition of dementia, one does the same for one's own self. In other words, by the perception and action of caring based on this affirmation of life through deep understanding and patience, the caregiver's own self may be reaffirmed.

One important factor in affirming the lives of persons with dementia is an understanding of the subjective experience of the condition of dementia. This has received increasing attention in the research literature of the recent past. The seminal volume in this regard—*The Person with Alzheimer's Disease: Pathways to Understanding the Experience*, edited by Phyllis Braudy Harris (2002)—is a much-needed compilation of studies exploring the subjective experiences of persons living with dementia. If we are to fully embrace a culture of dementia care in which the self is understood and honored, the person's own perspective on the frustrations, anxieties, and coping are critical. Also, books by persons with dementia, such as Thomas DeBaggio's *Losing My Mind: An Intimate Look at Life with Alzheimer's* (2002) and *When It Gets Dark: An Enlightened Reflection on Life with Alzheimer's* (2003) and Cary Henderson's *Partial View: An Alzheimer's Journal* (1998), provide valuable insights into what has been a secondhand perspective.

The challenges faced in dementia acquire a different set of dimensions on relocating to a long-term care facility. The long-term care setting, which is the context for many institutionalized elderly people, the majority of whom have some form of dementia, can be understood as integrating the related organizational policies and procedures, social climate, and physical environment (Moos and Lemke, 1994). These three dimensions of the setting are qualitatively different for residents who have had a lifetime of experience in homes and community environments. Philosophy of care, standards for admission, level of services, provision of privacy, personal control for residents, and flexibility of the programs—all affect the experience of the setting for the residents. Daily life revolves around a fairly structured routine of breakfast, lunch, dinner, bathing, and certain programmed activities. Frequently, the organizational culture in a nursing home creates a system in which individuals with chronic disease live their remaining days on acute care hospital models (J. N. Henderson, 1995).

The contrast between an institutional context and the places remembered from one's past becomes particularly salient for persons with dementia. In the early to middle stages of dementia, compromised cognitive functioning is an ever-present reality. The more enduring characteristics of self-identity are threatened by losses of physical and cognitive abilities and losses of places to which one was attached, creating a sense of self that is in turmoil. One tries to hold on to the identity one has known for years. At the same time, the changed socioenvironmental context offers the potential for recreation of the self. The task of conscious reflection on past experience can be a creative act in the sense that as we construct the pieces of the past in our minds, we are indeed reconstructing the content and context. Instead of the self-experience being *perceived* from a virtual computer screen of one's mind, it is *conceived* in an interpretive process. Memory can be viewed as a contraction of experience in a process of *sedimentation* (Ricoeur, 1992). In this process, temporally rooted life experiences are abstracted into memory, and in remembering we may "unpack" or "re-member" the sedimented dispositions to relive the past experience in the present time. Lived experiences are stored in memory not in a homogenous fashion but rather as a selective mechanism by which certain memories seem to have greater "retrievability" than others. Human remembering redeploys and expands the sedimented disposition of memories, and in this process of "unpacking" and "expanding," the creative aspect of self can recreate the past experience with fresh nuances and insights. As in the case of interpreting a literary text, all self-interpretations are dynamic and in evolution.

If the "I" aspect of self (James, 1890) is recognized as the creative and spontaneous dimension in the reminiscence process, remembering the personal past in a new perspective is an intriguing process. For the most part, this is a subconscious process in which all of us are constantly recreating our self-identities in subtle ways. The person I was ten years ago is not the same self I am today. This is a result of a natural process of redefinition and reshaping of one's self-identity. For a person with cognitive impairment, this process is much more affected by the cognitive-behavioral struggles, societal interactions, and the physical environment. Beyond the internal changes, the process is affected by the social perception of what is acceptable or not. The ways in which individuals in the social circle of a person with dementia accept, admonish, or put down a socially "unacceptable" behavior contribute to the person's process of self-recreation.

This notion relates to the idea of the social construction of the sense of self. Whatever we conceive as characterizing ourselves is in part a social and cultural construction. In other words, the definition of an "individual" —the social roles associated with and expected of an individual—shapes our construction of what we think of our self-identities. For example, if we as individuals acknowledge the social value of personal independence in our thoughts and actions, these features become part of our internal criteria of how we evaluate ourselves. It has been suggested that the memories associated with emotions are more accessible than other memories for people with dementia (Haight, 1991). Therefore, it can be hypothesized that *feelings* can be pivotal points in accessing past experiences. The emotions associated with remembered lived experiences can reshape the conception of self in more affective than rational terms. For example, in remembering the past a person can "feel" good by focusing on the positive life experiences rather than "rationalizing" what was achieved and what was not. Accepting the myriad events of life as part of a bigger picture can help one cope with unpleasant experiences and focus more on the larger context.

Feelings associated with places (e.g., strong emotional attachment to a particular home) may have a greater possibility of surfacing in remembering than relatively "neutral" experiences. The condition of "I *think,* therefore I am" as an accepted conceptualization of sense of self may be replaced by the created condition of "I *feel,* therefore I am." This avenue of rediscovery of the self holds much potential and challenge—particularly for adults with dementia whose sense of self is withering away. However, we can go beyond this level of self and recognize the essence of *being* that is underneath the self of feelings—the self that is simply *being.* At that level, self can be understood as "I *am,* therefore I am." This is the foundational shift that is needed in reframing the relational landscape with people with dementia.

CHAPTER TWO

Home

A Pathway to the Self in Dementia

It was the best place to be, thought Wilbur, this warm
delicious cellar with the garrulous geese, the changing
seasons, the heat of the sun, the passage of swallows, the
nearness of rats, the sameness of sheep, the love of spiders,
the smell of manure, and the glory of everything.

—*E. B. White*, Charlotte's Web *(1952)*

Home is a word that captures so much in our lives. Home is integral to our lived experiences. It is in our imagination and in our memories. The houses we grew up in, the neighborhoods where we played, the cities where we worked, are part and parcel of the mental landscape of lived experience that shapes and defines who we are, and as such they become deeply rooted in our memories. To be alive and conscious of one's life is at the fundamental level also to be aware of and interact with the places in one's life. As we live, work, and play, we do so in places around us, and through this process we give meaning to those places.

Among the various places that become meaningful for us, home is the single most significant one. Beyond meeting the need for a shelter, a true home is where we can be ourselves and be *at home*. Home sets the stage of our life experience; it is the psychological and emotional frame of reference from which we relate to all other places and life experiences. It is the space where we express ourselves and socially interact and where events of joy and sorrow take place. Home is where we grow old and become comfortable; it provides a setting where we can manage our daily lives in spite of physical frailty. Home is a reality defined by personal life experiences and, for some, a product of imagination. The never-seen home created in our longing, the faraway land that we have left behind, the land we may have never been to or may never visit, the garden that awaits as the abode in the hereafter—all live in imagination, as real as the places we inhabit now.

Because home is so central to our lives, memories of home are a powerful means for sustaining our sense of self. For people with dementia, memories of the places in their lives and the events, emotions, and experiences associated with those places can help provide continuity even as cognitive and communicative abilities dwindle. Reminiscence, especially reminiscence of home, can help caregivers and activity staff members better understand and care for persons with dementia. Helping older persons who have dementia recover a sense of self through memories of place can support, possibly even improve, quality of life in the face of the many losses associated with their disease.

Dementia's Challenges to the Self

Dementia leads to changes in mood, personality, and behavior, loss of social skills, restlessness, agitation, and progressive loss of motor skills, including the capacity for self-care. These multiple changes pose an increasing threat to personhood and result in, among other things, the loss of self-identity as we know it. In the early stages, people with dementia may feel acutely anxious and increasingly depressed as they become aware of failing memory and its associated problems, although memory for more distant places, times, events, and people may be relatively unimpaired compared with the ability to remember the recent past. In fact, in the condition of dementia (particularly Alzheimer disease), the person's reality reverts to the distant past. We often hear from caregivers that persons with dementia experience themselves as being in early childhood or young adulthood and talk about family or friends from those times in their lives. This shift in the perception of time is a critical aspect in acknowledging, affirming, and working with the temporal reality of the person with dementia.

At the same time, the transition to a nursing home means not only the loss of a familiar environment but also, in many instances, separation from the home to which the individual may have an emotional attachment. Moreover, the majority of long-term care facilities are places that afford few links with one's personal or cultural past. The typical care setting, in both its social and its physical aspects, reflects institutional policies and procedures as opposed to the personally meaningful place the resident has left behind. Facilities designed on the medical model of care can promote the adoption of generalized social roles, such as "old" and "sick," and deprive individuals of their familiar and meaningful environmental past.

Self and the Experience of Place

As humans trying to make sense of our world, we are incessantly involved in the process of bundling up information to make it easier to understand the multiplicity of our experience. We like to abstract things around us in mental constructions: a huge amount of water becomes an "ocean," large numbers of trees gathered together are a "forest," and so on. We give separate identities to these mental constructions in a process of *reification* (e.g., Csikszentmihalyi, 1993), attributing a sense of reality to abstractions in our imagination. Perhaps one of the most important of these abstractions is what we call the "self." In simple terms, our feelings, thoughts, emotions, impressions, and reactions distill into a reservoir of the self—shaping and building our identities as integrated entities. As we become conscious of the "self" and reflect on what makes up this self, we probably begin with a description of who we are (in terms of our emotions, intelligence, beliefs, values, etc.). These aspects of the self shape our human experience—that is, our human experience as it is shaped by our capacities to feel, to think, to believe, to comprehend, to act, and so on. From a temporal perspective, experience refers to the ever-accumulating subjective past from as far back as we can consciously remember. It is *what has been* that becomes the undeniable foundation of *who we are now.* If we are aware of what we have experienced and the emotions, thoughts, and beliefs that are associated with it, we can engage in a process of integration through which we discover and rediscover ourselves. As we remember our past life experiences, we have the ability to reflect on that experience from a relatively objective viewpoint and possibly make meaning of that experience. This conscious process of reflective remembering has the capacity to help us "own" our experiences in a meaningful way.

Places and things are important symbols of the self, cues to memories of important life experiences, and a means of maintaining, reviewing, and extending one's sense of self, especially in old age (Marcus, 1997; Csikszentmihalyi & Rochberg-Halton, 1981). Thus, environmental psychologists Proshansky, Fabian, and Kaminoff (1983) proposed that socialization of self is influenced not only by interactions with other people but also by relationships with various physical settings that define and structure everyday life. The authors maintain that what they call place identity "is a substructure of the self-identity of the person consisting of, broadly conceived, cognitions about the physical world in which the individual lives. These cognitions represent memories, ideas, feelings, attitudes, values, preferences, meanings, and conceptions of behavior and experience which relate to the variety and complexity of physical settings that define the day-to-day existence of every human being. At the core of such physical environment related cognitions is the 'environmental past' of the person" (Proshansky et al., 1983, p. 59).

The nature and content of life experiences across several dimensions contribute in creating our self-identities. Our experience of the world occurs in overlapping social, organizational, psychological, and physical contexts. Individuals have psychological characteristics, intentions, desires, and goals and interact with others in a social context that is defined by particular norms, values, and attitudes. Often, these interactions take place in organizational contexts—such as care facilities—governed by explicit or implicit philosophies, missions, policies, and regulations.

The physical environment is perhaps the most frequently overlooked of these dimensions. Experiences take place in certain physical settings, be they natural or built environments. To *be* is to exist somewhere, and to exist somewhere means to be in some *place*. Bodily human experience cannot occur "out of place" any more than it can happen "out of time." Consequently, memories of these experiences become anchored in certain places—for example, the memories of our youth that are tied to the house we grew up in or the secret places of childhood and adolescence, or those of adulthood that are tied to the house in which we raised our children. Memories of these places are as much a part of the experience as any other dimensions that we recall.

Place and the Aging Self

What is the experience of place like for older people? Traditionally, the field of environment and aging focused more on the sensory than the experiential aspects of place. This is a consequence both of the intellectual tradition that has emphasized a view of humans as adaptive organisms reacting to stimuli and of the functional reality of the physical and sensory limitations that accompany old age. This research has looked at the difficulties older people encounter in navigating and functioning in their environment. Thus, the majority of the studies of home and housing have focused on quantifiable features, such as objective environmental features of the home, distance from key resources, safety, environmental barriers, and building type. Outcome measures typically have been well-being or satisfaction. A few naturalistic or qualitative studies have taken a more individually oriented approach, seeking to isolate the discrete psychosocial processes by which older persons form and maintain links and attachments to their homes. For example, Rubinstein (1989) described how older people use social-, person-, and body-centered processes to facilitate the connection of self to the home environment. This approach views the home as existing at the nexus of individual and collective meaning, blending individuals' unique personal histories with the cultural icon of safety and security.

Only recently have we begun to explore the affective or emotional processes, the symbolic constructions, the phenomenology of places, and the relationship of this environmental experience in self-definition. There are suggestions that people act proactively on the physical environment, selecting and adapting their surroundings to enhance competence and the achievement of desired goals; in other words, not only does the physical environment shape life experience and identity, but also the reverse is true. Thus, environment can be seen as an integral part of lived experience; consequently, environmental memories could be cues for remembering past experience. Three of the most significant of these new ways of thinking about environment and aging are the concepts of attachment to place, insidedness, and continuity.

Attachment to place—that is, the phenomenon of people's emotional and cultural attachment to environmental settings, such as homes—has received considerable attention as an attempt to understand the subjective meaning of environments. Researchers Rubinstein and Parmelee (1992) suggested a model of place identity in late life that attempts to integrate both collective and individual factors with physical, personal, and social factors. Importantly, they argue that it is on the individual level that space is given meaning. The spaces and the physical environment in a home gain meaning through an individual's experiences in those spaces. For example, the activities that take place in an individual's living room, including social interactions, family events, and the like, make that space memorable for the person. Or the backyard garden where someone has spent hours gardening has a special place in the person's life, developing an emotional attachment for that person.

Places, like homes, do not have inherent meaning. We give them meaning, or rather we *create* the meaning of places in our minds based on the meaning of our life events. This phenomenon of attachment to place can happen to public places as well. For example, an individual's experience of a plaza or a park is influenced by his or her subjective preference, intentions, and past place experiences, as well as by the social values, norms, and symbolism of that public place. Attachment to place can be understood as an outcome of how well any particular place facilitates goals and activities. In other words, attachment to place can be a function of the extent to which the environment supports one's needs and preferences. For example, an older adult may become intimately familiar with a home where he or she has lived for many years. Even if the home has objective shortcomings (e.g., lack of adequate space in the kitchen), it might be able to support the individual's functions because the familiarity works as a buffer between behavioral competence and the environment. Obviously, as an individual's physical condition declines over time, the physical environment may not be able to support daily activities.

One way to understand how we develop this relationship with places over time is the model of place experience proposed by Weisman and colleagues (2000). This model suggests that we experience places through perception, cognition, action, affect, and meaning. We perceive the environment through our senses (perception), understand or make sense of that environment based on our past experience and present goals or needs (cognition), and perform activities as appropriate (action). This process may have a component that relates to our preference and emotions (affect) and one that relates to significance (meaning). These aspects of place experience are fused in forming the core of place experience that over time develops into "sense-of-self-in-place"—an intangible part of self-identity, which reflects the experiential aspects that relate to, and as a result become part of, the self.

A growing body of work has pointed out that personal experience gives meaning to places and contributes to self-identity (e.g., Rowles & Chaudhury, 2005). Environmental gerontologist Graham Rowles introduced the concept of *insideness* (1983), which is particularly illuminating in this discussion. Briefly, insideness refers to the taken-for-granted aspects of lived experience. Rowles identifies three aspects of insideness: physical, social, and autobiographical. *Physical insideness* relates to the experiential familiarity with the environment one develops over time that results in an implicit awareness of the physical features of an environment—for example, knowing the exact location of a light switch in one's bedroom or the layout of items on a given grocery aisle. *Social insideness* reflects the social relationships, patterns of interdependence, and general social milieu that become integrated with place experience—for example, the familiarity of social interactions with well-known people in the neighborhood. Over time, a particular locale develops a social rhythm and ambiance that contributes to the creation of a sense of social awareness. The third aspect of insideness, *autobiographical insideness,* is particularly relevant and illuminating in helping us understand the context of place experience and the aging self. The process involves projecting a sense of self into places of significance and creating a place that reminds one of one's identity. In this process of transfusion of self with the physical environment, individuals become emotionally attached to particular places. Rowles (1983) argues that this aspect of insideness is particularly internal and is rarely overtly communicated. It also involves places from a past that has, over the life span, shaped the contour of one's identity.

Environmental gerontologist Boschetti (1984) identified three themes linked with self-identity in old age: connection, caring, and continuity. *Connection* is the psychological bond with people, places, or events created by shared experience or personal associations. *Caring* refers to concern with the well-being of the people and places with which one has such bonds. *Continuity* characterizes the attachment of self to specific places. Identification with special places remembered from one's past or experienced continuously over much of one's life gives continuity to one's sense of self and establishes a meaningful core in our relationship with the places in our lives.

These conceptualizations of place as *spaces that have been given meaning through personal, group, or cultural processes* vary in scale and scope, in focusing on tangible versus symbolic characteristics, and in their emphasis on present or past. Yet all begin with geographical locale—the physical locations, characteristics, and sensory and perceptually distinguishing features that identify one place from other places. And all take "place" to signify meaningful identification with the locale beyond mere physical environmental characteristics, such as experience of significant events, sense of cultural heritage, sense of rootedness, and functional dependence. Each envisions the experience of place as processes of confluence of individual emotions and characteristics of place, emphasizing the central role of the self and its nature as a repository of place experience. Each emphasizes that the experience of place in relation to self is subjective and idiosyncratic. Likewise, each argues that places are affectively redefined in remembering, reminiscence, and social interaction. The meaning and relative importance of any attribute of place may shift with life experiences in a dynamic relationship that is often overlooked if we focus on discrete geographical locales or events.

Reminiscence and the Aging Self

Although the process of looking back and understanding our selfhood is one in which we engage across our life span, it becomes more relevant as we grow older, as a natural process of "summing up," to make meaning out of our experienced lives. The realization that life will come to an end effects a shift in how we look at time so that we come to measure it by how much is left rather than by how much has elapsed since birth. As we age, the prospect of new events and experiences becomes restricted, a consequence of the duration of a natural life span. At this later stage in life, reminiscence about the past can become fairly common; indeed, in the popular mind, old age and reminiscence are intimately linked. However, the general tendency is to take reminiscence for granted as a mundane feature of old age rather than to explore these wonderfully rich memories as a source of self-continuity and personal growth for the older person.

In the activities of remembering and reminiscing we are continually structuring, maintaining, and reconstructing our self-identities. Remembering, be it a subconscious or automatic recollection of what we are supposed to do the next moment or a conscious recollection of what we did last year, is universal, a natural process occurring in different intensities across the life span. The frequency and intensity of reminiscence increase with aging, primarily because of increasing awareness of one's mortality and a shift in time orientation. Remembering and reminiscence help us maintain our self-identity. The capacity to make the past vivid, preferably in the presence of a sympathetic listener, can be one of the key resources older adults use to maintain psychological health. This theme of self-preservation lies behind most reminiscence work carried out in institutional settings, in which cognitively intact persons are encouraged to see their life experience as something to be valued and shared with others. Similarly, maintaining self-esteem has been a focus of research that has tried to establish empirically the value of reminiscence—for example, studies of the relationships between reminiscence and adjustment in elderly people undergoing relocation (e.g., Rowles, 1993; Lieberman and Tobin, 1983).

The value of reminiscence as a means of maintaining self-esteem and morale increases in the face of losses or critical transitions in one's life. The loss of parental, marital, and vocational roles and functions that accompany aging may bring a lessening of one's sense of self unless some countervailing processes take place. Relocation to an institution or even to another house entails leaving behind the familiar, the place in which one has invested the self, for an uncertain and unfamiliar environment (as both a physical and a social context).

Relevant to the issue of reminiscence as a mechanism for self-preservation is the debate in the gerontological literature about whether there is change or stability, flexibility or rigidity, in personality functioning in late life. The empirical evidence is inconclusive, though some studies suggest that there is greater rigidity in personality characteristics as persons grow older. On the one hand, the more observable aspects of personality—those that have to do with sociability, interpersonal behaviors, and lifestyle—generally tend to show stability and continuity over the life span. On the other hand, the inner functioning of the personality seems to change in old age, suggesting that there may be increased saliency of the inner life and introspection in old age. This introspection includes more focusing of thought and feeling on inner issues in relation to external or environmental issues; many of these inner processes deal with sorting out experiences, persons, values, and things that are central to the self (Sherman, 1995).

Reminiscence in Dementia Care

For older adults in residential care, assisted living, or adult day programs, reminiscing about significant places from the past can offer a powerful means of remembering one's life course. To the extent that care and activities are based on institutional values, policies, and procedures, residents or clients face the potential of losing or at least compromising their self-identity. Nursing homes in particular are places that stand in contrast with the community settings where residents (or prospective residents) have lived all their lives. These facilities symbolize a withdrawal from community and the institutionalization of physical dependency. In general, in the nursing home, where the organizational and collective approaches of caregiving often dominate the social and physical environments, there is limited opportunity for self-expression. Institutional policies and routines largely overtake self-identity and personal meaning, creating compromised physical and social environments in terms of personal preference, values, and lifestyle.

In the face of the erosion of the sense of self experienced by persons with dementia, reminiscence can provide the context of events, places, and people from the past to which the individual with dementia might relate. Given the potential strength of reminiscence in caregiving for people with dementia, one might expect to find a substantial body of research in this avenue of intervention. In reality, there have been few empirical studies addressing reminiscence for people with dementia. In general, however, those studies have demonstrated that reminiscence has a positive influence, in terms of improved communication between residents and staff, increased self-esteem, reduced agitation, and higher ego-integrity, for cognitively impaired elderly people in residential care (Gibson, 2004; Gotell et al., 2002).

Reminiscence can play a role in helping caregivers fulfill the goal of providing high-quality care. To ensure the quality of care, one must understand the subjective meaning of quality of life for residents. Lawton (1983) spoke of "the good life" as involving four essential features of the environment and other determinants of well-being in older adults' lives: behavioral competence, psychological well-being, perceived quality of life, and the objective environment. These four features interrelate to give form and shape to behavior, environment, and experience. To create a meaningful living environment in the nursing home, we need to understand these sectors not in isolation but in an integrative fashion that resembles real-life experience for the residents (Lawton, 1983). This process of understanding should begin in grasping the unique identities of the residents as reflected through their personal pasts and in recognizing and appreciating their life histories. Who are they as individuals? What are their values, preferences, beliefs, and attitudes? What are the places in which they lived? What are their life experiences associated with those places? Kitwood's (1997) pioneering "person-centered" care approach emphasized the importance of knowing the life history of the person with dementia. Personal life history provides the foundation for understanding the person behind the condition of dementia. Kitwood aptly pointed out, "We are learning now that much can be done to maintain identity in the face of cognitive impairment. Two things seem to be essential. The first is knowing in some detail about each individual's life history; even if a person cannot hold on to his or her own narrative identity, due to loss of memory, it can still be held by others. The second is empathy, through which it is possible to respond to a person as Thou, in the uniqueness of his or her being" (p. 84).

For people with dementia, who have impaired short-term memory and relatively intact long-term memory, reconnecting with the personal past makes intuitive sense. Personal memories are more likely to be accessible than memories of impersonal events. Because personally meaningful memories are reconstructed on a number of occasions during a person's life, they are more likely to have affective associations, which enhance their memorability. Through the act of remembering, the individual with dementia may be able to reexperience the past, including the emotions associated with the place or event remembered. An example of the potential of reminiscence to enhance communication for persons with dementia is found in a study by Moss and colleagues (2002). This study explored reminiscence as a potential medium of communication between the nursing staff and residents with Alzheimer disease. The study suggested that participating in reminiscence is a way for residents to offset some of the losses that come with Alzheimer disease. Although persons with dementia often have difficulty communicating on the cognitive level, Moss and colleagues found that when study participants reminisced about "heartfelt, memorable events, their language appeared more fluent" (p. 38). The study also suggested that exchanges during reminiscence sessions can facilitate the building of trust and "may help staff in understanding how certain events have helped shape patients' personalities" (p. 42).

Brooker and Duce (2000) compared individuals involved in simple reminiscence therapy using "multisensory props" (objects and photographs) with those involved in group activities (such as crafts or games) and with residents enjoying "unstructured time." Using Dementia Care Mapping (Bradford Dementia Group, 1997), an observational tool designed to "evaluate the quality of care from the point of view of the person with dementia," these researchers compared participants' levels of well-being while involved in one of the three groups: reminiscence therapy (RT), structured group activity (GA), and unstructured time (UT). Brooker and Duce's (2000) data showed that participants involved in the RT group displayed a higher level of well-being during the activity than did participants in the other activities. They attribute this improvement to the fact that reminiscence sessions were designed to enable participants with varying levels of cognition to participate to the extent that they were able or comfortable.

As practiced in dementia care settings, individual reminiscence work is rare (e.g., Gibson, 1994); group reminiscence sessions have been the norm to date. A typical reminiscence group is a structured or semistructured activity in which the leader assists and guides the group members in recalling previous experiences and facilitates the group's affirmation of the value of these experiences. Themes and props are used as adjuncts for reminiscence sessions. The *theme* is the topic of discourse and discussion —chosen by the leader or by members—that serves as a unifying, dominant idea for the session. The purpose of the theme includes providing structure to the group and helping to reduce the anxiety of the members. A theme is most effective if it catches the interest of group members and increases their participation as well as the depth and breadth of their recollections. General themes that are typically used to elicit reminiscence include food preparation, music, occupations, relationships, fashion, travel, and weather. *Props* may include a variety of items used to trigger memories of events, persons, or places, such as personal artifacts, memorabilia, visual aids, dolls, fishing gear, and so on. Props can be particularly helpful in providing sensory stimulation or eliciting memories in persons with dementia.

The selection of themes or props may seem like a simple matter, but participants' ability to recollect, as well as the depth and breadth of their recollections, may depend very much on the appropriateness of the themes or props. Moreover, for people with dementia a theme that relates to the personal past, with verbal and visual prompts from the individual's past, can be more effective than a generic theme (Chaudhury, 2003). Reminiscence with people who have dementia requires a sensitive approach. As with any other group, there will be individual differences, and not all older people enjoy reminiscing. Moreover, people with dementia often have difficulty making sense of their world, particularly when faced with a new situation, and without careful planning, reminiscence may generate anxiety in them. Sensitive issues, such as the nature of family relationships or finances, should generally be avoided in group work but may be handled in one-on-one reminiscence. In the event of highly emotional recollection, the person may need psychological support both during and after the session.

Remembering Home

Despite evidence of the therapeutic potential of reminiscence for persons with dementia, little effort has been directed toward understanding the content, themes, and meaning of reminiscence. For example, no study to date has looked at the probable variation in recollection across different topics of reminiscence. Remembering the personal past may provide the continuity that is personally meaningful for persons with dementia. In the unfamiliar social and physical environment of a nursing home, recalling past events, activities, and places may provide psychological support to one's sense of self-worth. Although there is anecdotal support that experience of place "creeps into" recollections (Gibson, 1994), the potential of using place as an explicit theme for reminiscence remains unexplored. In the unfamiliar environment of a nursing home, remembering significant past places presents a promising therapeutic process and may make life a little more bearable for cognitively impaired residents.

In particular, remembrance of past homes can help in redefining aspects of the self in the current changed environmental context. The construction of the past could be seen as a emotional process, rather than a neutral and mechanical process. Beyond the nostalgic recollection of the past, guided reminiscence sessions can be a consciously engaging process for the older adult. This process can be mindful and dynamic as new aspects are brought in and familiar experiences are reinterpreted in a fresh light, and in this process the self is *rediscovered*. The prospect of rediscovering the self is particularly intriguing for people with dementia. The potential of reminiscence as a process of reconstructing self-identity in older adults is acknowledged conceptually (Kitwood, 1997), as is the role of places in contributing to the evolving self (Gibson, 1994). But these issues have not been explored empirically among older adults with dementia. At the same time, the potential influence of a nursing home environment on stimulating (or failing to stimulate) residents' environmental memories must be acknowledged. For example, the opportunity to walk in a garden at a nursing home may trigger a resident's memories of gardening at her home. For a resident who lived all his life in urban locations, a rural nursing home may not be a stimulating environment.

Reminiscence about places with persons who have dementia also has considerable potential, largely unexplored, as a methodology for staff development. Understanding individuals in the context of their former social lives, in their homes and communities, has the potential to reduce the strong institutional demarcation of social roles as "residents" or "clients" vis-à-vis "caregivers." Those who provide care for people with dementia in institutional settings are often accustomed to labeling these residents as "confused." By reducing residents to their stage of disease and observed symptoms, this fails to acknowledge them as persons, as *selves* with pasts and memories. It is crucial that caregivers have the knowledge of the residents as persons with preferences, attitudes, and, more important, life histories. Behavioral and communication difficulties could be better understood if we relate to the person with dementia through these avenues instead of isolating the challenges in their own right. The immediate necessity of "managing" behaviors may inhibit caregivers from listening and empathizing appropriately. Too often, when interactions with residents are accompanied by expressions of emotion, such as tears or sadness, caregivers tend to change the subject, try to distract the resident, or physically withdraw. Reminiscence can help fill the need for a process that would enable the staff to know about residents as *individuals*—persons who have unique life histories, come from diverse backgrounds, have their own place experiences—and so to empathize with them. As staff members become more knowledgeable about the personal life histories of residents, there is a potential for increased tolerance, understanding, and empathy. This can contribute to more meaningful and rewarding interactions between staff and residents, which in turn may have a positive effect on staff attitude and job satisfaction. Although the latter outcomes are relatively indirect, they would have important implications for residents' quality of life. That is, reminiscence can be a tool to improve the nursing home experience for both residents *and* staff.

CHAPTER THREE

Home as a Setting for Lived Experience

We lived on Waverly Place, in a warm, clean, two-bedroom flat that sat above a small Chinese bakery specializing in steamed pastries and dim sum. In the early morning, when the alley was still quiet, I could smell fragrant red beans as they were cooked down to a past sweetness. By daybreak, our flat was heavy with the odor of fried sesame balls and sweet curried crescents. From my bed, I would listen as my father got ready for work, then locked the door behind him, one-two-three clicks.

—*Amy Tan*, Rules of the Game *(1989)*

How do homes become a part of our memories? As Amy Tan's eloquent recollection of her childhood home illustrates, often it is the everyday activities and mundane details of life that help us remember the places. In the previous chapter we saw how place and memories of place play an important role in shaping—and sustaining—our sense of self. Memories of home, especially, are part of our self-identity. But, as we also saw, the potential role of these memories and connections with the places of our personal pasts, unique to each individual, in the care of for persons with dementia has for the most part not been the focus of research. In this chapter I draw on my own research with residents and family members to address that gap. In particular, I draw on interviews with 13 individuals with dementia and members of their families that were carried out in four care facilities in Wisconsin to develop the concept of "home story," a place-based, home-related biographical sketch that synthesizes a resident's memories of home and that might serve as a tool for guided reminiscence.

I began by asking family members about memories their loved ones had shared with them of the loved one's connections with places, such as childhood homes, the places they'd lived as young adults, and so on. The recollections participants shared with me reveal that memories of home are complex and layered. Most of the family members I talked with were close relatives, such as daughters, sons, or siblings of the residents with dementia. For siblings, many of the residents' childhood memories would overlap with their own, while the daughters and sons recounted stories they had heard from their parents or described pictures or artifacts they had seen. Several key themes emerged in these conversations, and a few themes were specific to childhood. Place-based recollections of childhood centered around themes of belonging to a place and place anchors outside the home. Memories of adult years revealed themes of place as process and attachment to home.

Belonging to a Place

We can describe ourselves in terms of multiple aspects—age, gender, occupation, family, house, city, and so on—which provide resources that help each of us create our self-identity; in this process of creation, the aspects become constructs and realities to which we "belong." Carl Jung (1989) pointed out the innate need of the self to express itself in the surrounding, to be part of others, and to make others part of oneself. From childhood through our adult years, our experiences with particular others, in particular places, play an important role in creating a sense of belonging.

Family members of persons with dementia noted that their loved ones' most frequent recollections after the diagnosis of dementia were of childhood times and places, as if those memories are the foundation of who they are and how they prefer to "remember" themselves. The sense of belonging was not expressed exclusively in association with childhood places. However, places from childhood were prevalent in all of the recollections, distinguishing them from memories of later years. Even when the recollections involved unpleasant incidents from childhood years, families talked about understanding the person as having a sense of acceptance, as though time had healed the painful aspects of the memories and all that remained were things to be treasured. The way family members spoke about their loved ones and the memories loved ones had shared with them suggested that the childhood home and the sense of creating one's own world were salient features in the person's sense of belonging to a place.

In the following case studies, names and other identifying details (e.g., home address) have been changed to preserve confidentiality.

Childhood Home

Some of the strongest memories of place are associated with the places of childhood. Childhood is the time of growing up, of becoming conscious of one's ego-self, of differentiating between self and other. Just as we develop relationships with others around us, so do we create relationships with places, and they become embedded in our childhood memories. Special events related to nature, holidays, or other activities can make a place memorable. For instance, Julia, who had lived in a nursing home for the past three years, visited her grandparents' farm in Nebraska. Her daughter recalled how Julia spoke about her childhood on the farm, and especially an incident involving a lightning storm that occurred there once. The lightning was memorable and was connected with Julia's memory of her grandparents' farm. As Julia's daughter recounted:

And one time while she was in her grandparents' home in Nebraska, there was a big lightning storm. And I think they had just done something with the electricity there—they had just gotten it or something, and lightning did strike. She does remember being in bed that night with the lightning and something with the light.

Another resident, Maria, had been in a care facility for a few years. Her daughter spoke about her mother based on a combination of a family photograph and what she had heard from Maria:

I've seen pictures of the house that she was born in. Her father was a caretaker for a fairgrounds in Menomonie and so they lived on this fairgrounds, in a house on the fairgrounds.

Sheila's nephew had firsthand experience of his aunt's childhood farm, and he recalled the home, describing the physical characteristics of the house, along with the lack of such amenities as running water and electricity. Such additional functional aspects might perhaps be recalled and shared in the context of the striking contrast with the situation in one's present home. Changes in circumstances can be considered self-producing prompts for remembering. If what used to be is no more, or is very different, the associated memories seem to "stand out" by default. Sheila's childhood was characterized by hard work on the farm and by simplicity, as is revealed in her nephew's memories:

Her childhood home was a single-family, three-bedroom, wood-frame structure, without plumbing, running water, or electricity. Toilet facilities were outdoor privies; water was all carried in from a well. Light was provided by candles and lanterns. Simple things, such as soap, were homemade, no store-bought stuff. I remember the house and, being a child, found no particular discomfort physical or mental while there.

Unique episodes can make a place memorable. Holiday events, special occasions, or something out of the ordinary becomes engraved in memory along with the place. The element of surprise can be a catalyst in making a place special. Perhaps this is especially true for events in childhood. One story that Maria had repeatedly shared with her daughter was the first time she saw electric lights on a Christmas tree in her home. The vividness of her memory of that event comes through in her daughter's recollection:

I'm not sure if this was in Menomonie or in Racine when they lived in Racine, but the first electric lights on the Christmas tree that her parents surprised them with . . . And she'd say, "I can still picture it." They had [them] go in the other room, and it was a big living room and dining room, and the Christmas tree was in the corner. And they always had candles on the tree. And here they brought them into the room, she and her brother, into the living room—maybe they had to close their eyes—and then all of a sudden they turned on those lights on that Christmas tree, and they were just in awe. So that was a wonderful experience. And . . . when she talks about it, she has that room, you know, pictured.

This illustrates how one particular event from childhood can become deeply etched in our memories. The fact that Maria had recollected that childhood experience with her daughter repeatedly indicates the poignancy of that memory.

Creating One's Own World

Children will play wherever they are, and in their play they innovate and create. Playing with friends, imagining their own little homes, and having a carefree time are part of the process in which places become meaningful and memories are created, as the recollections offered by residents and family members showed. Joyce grew up on a farm, and her play area included the farm and a nearby woods. In addition to the work she used to do on the family farm, there also seemed to be time for play and a sense of joy. Her daughter recalled Joyce's talking about playing with her sisters on the farm:

> *She talked about the few dolls that she had . . . 'cause it was a poor family, and how she and her sisters used to go to the woods, to the wooded area, and they made houses there and played with their dolls and created their own little world. There was a spring not far from where their farm was located, the farm buildings, and she used to go there to the spring and that's where they played. They had a lot of fun there.*

Julia's memorable play moments were in a home and neighborhood in the town of New London, Wisconsin. She had good friends in the neighborhood and talked about them when she recounted stories of playtime to her daughter. Julia's daughter talked about her mother's bedroom in her childhood home as she narrated an incident she had heard from her mother:

> *I'm sure she had her bedroom upstairs. She used to talk about a friend, a girlfriend, who lived next door and the houses were fairly close to each other. And I think their bedroom windows must have been facing each other. Because she said that, at one point in their growing-up years, they had strung up a little pulley thing between the two windows with the ropes, and they would pass messages back and forth on this pulley thing.*

These activities happened in the children's own carefree world, one created by imagination, creativity, and innocence and remembered in later years. Such childhood activities go beyond "child's play" in their power to stay in memory into very late life.

Place Anchors outside the Home

If home is the central place that embodies and anchors memories of lived experience, there are other places that shape, mediate, and anchor place memories. Places such as the neighborhoods and cities where we have lived or spent meaningful time are often also salient parts of our life experience. In discussions with residents and families, memories of these places emerged as they talked about their homes. Indeed, for home to be truly meaningful, there had to be "other" places. The significance of home is related to these places in the neighborhood and the city: workplace, grocery store, park, café, bookshop, and so on. They are also the public spaces where one meets others. Activities such as casual social interactions in a coffee shop, community gatherings in a town hall, group meetings for a cause, or simply sitting alone in a public square give one the opportunity to be part of the collective. These places become important parts of our lived experiences and, in turn, of our memories, anchoring experiences outside of the realm of one's home. In the memories recounted by residents and family members, anchors outside the home included neighborhood life, city as collective, and natural context.

Neighborhood Life

For these residents, neighborhood was a significant part of remembering the home of their early adulthood. In a natural sequence from remembering the home itself, they shared memories of the physical characteristics of neighborhoods they had lived in, the neighborly interactions, and the community activities. This identifies the importance of the physicality of places in residents' recollections as reported by family members. Not only did the physical proximity of neighborhood homes and neighbors play a distinct role in residents' lives, but also the neighbors' homes played a role in being recollected as significant places after the home.

Neighbors are essential ingredients of a neighborhood. However, one's sense of community or neighborliness can vary greatly, depending on various issues. In general, the neighborhoods recollected by the residents or family members interviewed brought up a positive image of neighbors. Interactions and sometimes friendships with neighbors contributed to remembering neighborhoods. For example, Maria's daughter recollected her mother's neighbors (who were her own childhood neighbors) firsthand and alluded to neighbors as something that made the neighborhood pleasant:

> There was all kinds of neighbors. We had ones right next to us who were very, very kindly, an older couple, very kindly. Above them was a family, and my mother was close, made good friends with the woman. There was the old biddy next to us. She was the German lady that was meticulous. So there was the whole variety of neighbors. It was a very pleasant neighborhood and, as I said, very convenient for anything that was needed, especially because we didn't have a car. You had everything right in the area.

Julia's daughter recalled her mother's dislike of the neighborhood in California where she lived for a short time with her husband and daughter. Julia had lived in a dense neighborhood in Wisconsin where the houses were closely spaced; the widely separated houses of a California neighborhood were unfamiliar to her. She felt that people were psychologically distant from one another, in contrast to her pleasant, neighborly memories of people back in Wisconsin. Also, she talked about the unpredictability of neighbors who were perhaps different from her earlier experience of neighbors and neighborhoods. Her daughter presents Julia's case:

> If you talk about neighborhoods and homes, it seems as though the homes that she lived in that were close together were the ones that she probably liked. Most of them were close together. And for other reasons, she may not have liked the one in California. But those houses were farther apart. Then again, it was a whole different atmosphere there. And I wouldn't say she was very happy in California. Neither was my dad, for that matter. That house [in California] would not be one that she would remember fondly. But it was a glamorous house, in California. You know, in El Porto. It was palm trees

and all this stuff. The lady down the street had her hair a different color every week. If it was St. Patrick's Day, it was green. Very shallow living, and they didn't like that. So they didn't stay there very long, obviously, from '60 to '63, about two years that they lived there.

Joyce grew up in a rural area in Wisconsin and went to a one-room school. Her school days were recollected by her son:

She went to a one-room school, grades one through eight. It was called the Clausen School. It was a little country school, and it basically was just an immediate farm neighborhood. It was approximately, I may just say, about three miles from her home. And under normal conditions, she walked to school and home every day. She told us all the different little adventures that took place on the way to or coming back from school.

In general, school was a well-liked place. For residents who grew up in rural areas, walking to school was part of enjoying time on their own. Talking with friends, feeling safe on familiar routes, occasionally stopping at certain spots—all these made the walks interesting and memorable. It was a time of their own, a transition time between home and school. Time at home typically was spent in play, helping out, doing things with family, whereas time at school was mostly spent in studying. Walking to the school and back created a time when the children were by themselves outside the purview of home or school—a time that gave a each person sense of freedom and of being trusted by adults.

City as Collective

Beyond one's neighborhood, the larger context of the city can define and shape memories of the places we share with others—places that provide the context for one's sense of being part of the collective. In the memories recalled by residents and family members, places in cities where they had lived emerged as a source of romantic fascination and a salient context for memories of home. For example, Brenda loved Milwaukee, especially the lake. She moved to Milwaukee in her later years to live with her daughter. To Brenda, the city of Milwaukee meant Lake Michigan. Although she did not have her own home in the city and had not grown up there, the city had its place in her memory because of her love of the lake. Her daughter shared:

> My mother loves Milwaukee, always loved it. She loves Lake Michigan. She calls it her ocean. She wrote poems and stories about the lake.

For Janet, memories of Milwaukee were tied to exploration and moving about. As a young adult she moved around the city with her friends. It became a pastime for her and a memory that she had shared with her nephew. Janet's nephew remembered for his aunt:

> She used to go to concerts when she was much younger. She'd go with different girlfriends or her sisters. In fact, they were fond of walking all around the town, because rather than spend the few pennies it took to ride the streetcar, they would save their money so they could buy ice cream or go to a movie. And they would walk, even late at night. Aunt Janet told me often how this walking about in the city became a sort of passion for her and how she found that exciting, to find out new places in the city.

Association with a place based on cultural identity can reflect an individual's experience of a city as part of a desire to belong to a collective. In a somewhat different way from Brenda or Janet, Sheila liked Milwaukee for its cultural/ethnic associations. Although she had grown up on a farm, once she moved to Milwaukee, she came to appreciate the cultural connection and chose to live in the city for all her adult years. The language and culture that were part of her self-identity provided the basis of commonality between her and the city of Milwaukee. Sheila's nephew talked about the contrasting urban versus rural life his aunt had led and pointed out how her preference for city life in adult years was a result of a natural affinity:

> Her addresses were always central city—within walking distance of "downtown." From the isolation of childhood, she seems to have gravitated to the hustle of central city. I have a hunch she was ethnic-oriented. Milwaukee at that time was a German city. She spoke the language, was raised in a German culture/custom environment. It seems only natural, in retrospect, that a late-teen-aged girl would be drawn to a place wherein she was most

comfortable. For her, Milwaukee was the place to live. She spent her entire
adult life in that city. During her younger years, the only language she used,
at home, in school, socially, and in church, was German.

Place as Process

A place becomes meaningful to the self through processes that involve, among other things, human aspirations, emotions, and expectations. Place is not a static end product of emotions and nostalgia, but also a dynamic and evolving process in which geographic locales acquire personal significance. Understood as process, place cannot be reduced to space or time, although these dimensions are part of our inner landscape. As process, place encompasses an ongoing dynamic in which the significance and meaning of place are continually renewed and regenerated.

Residents' and family members' memories of home revealed four key attributes of place as process: creating the texture of daily life, expressing one's self, raising a family, and threading memories from generation to generation. As we inhabit, act, and exist in places, we create and recreate who we are—to ourselves and to others. Being in a place is not to be static but to move around, to perform activities, and, more subtly, to grow into one's self. And in this process of growth, places play an integral part by giving us the opportunity to express ourselves, to change the place around us, and to be part of a collective memory.

Creating the Texture of Daily Life

The concept of place as process emerges when we think of how our memories of place and our sense of self are saturated with the experience of doing particular things in particular places—perhaps especially with the memory of routines we are hardly aware of as we carry them out every day. We tend to remember better the activities and celebrations that are spaced apart in time, like Christmas or New Year's Eve—annual activities that we plan, anticipate, celebrate, and then start planning again for next year. These activities or rituals gain added importance through the collective meaning that we ascribe to them. Celebrating a holiday and participating in the associated activities (e.g., going to see fireworks on the Fourth of July) have both personal and explicitly shared collective significance. Through these activities, we make some places memorable that are shared by others, such as a plaza where the city's Christmas tree is placed or a war memorial in honor of slain soldiers.

However, on an individual level, the daily activities—the unconscious routine of doing things that is an integral part of daily life—make places personally meaningful. Waking up, making coffee, getting ready for work, returning home from work, preparing meals, gardening, washing clothes, and so on are all part of people's everyday activities in the home. These activities do not require a lot of planning, yet they take place (for the most part) in predictable patterns in predictable places within the home. Cooking is done in the kitchen, morning coffee is drunk at the kitchen table, and a book is read in the living room; most of the activities take place in certain locations. These activities happening in the same places at the same times form the texture of daily life. In general, we take these everyday "rituals" for granted, carrying on with them without much notice; nevertheless, they give meaning and structure to our lives.

Linda's niece remembered Linda's gardening and how important that activity was to her. For Linda, it went beyond taking care of the flowers and raising vegetables; many after-gardening activities were tied to her work in the garden. She regularly and diligently canned produce to reduce her dependency on grocery store produce. These activities contributed to her pride in homemaking and taking care of the family, as her niece recalled:

> *My aunt had a large garden, which meant that she did a lot of canning garden vegetables, and would purchase a lot of fruit and preserve [it]. This was a significant part of her life. She would put up enough food that we hardly had to go to a grocery store in the early days. And I suppose that those would be significant things to her because she always took a lot of pride in doing those things. They were very, very special for her.*

Cooking was a common activity of many residents' adult years. It was often taken seriously, and, naturally, the activity was done in the kitchen. Kitchens figured prominently in recollections of activities that took place in people's homes. The residents and family members I interviewed represent the cohort who were, for the most part, homemakers. They took pride in keeping up with household activities, and their kitchens were symbolic of their territorial control over their houses. Julia's daughter remembered that her mother liked cooking, household work, and local social activities. For Maria, these "rituals" helped structure her daily life and home activities. In her daughter's recollection:

> My mother was a good cook. She used to like to spend a lot of time in the kitchen. I think the kitchen was the first room that she checked out when they were checking out new places. And she cooked very good meals... And she liked doing floral arrangements. She was in a neighborhood garden club or whatever for some years. And the altar guild in church. Those kinds of things she liked to do. And she liked to entertain small groups at a time. I don't think she liked big parties.

For Helena, everyday activities gained meaning in her routines of doing things at her home. She carried out her household rituals like clockwork. For her, a strict pattern of activities was the only way of doing things. As a family friend described her:

> [Helena] had routines that were just amazing. And in fact, I think that's part of why she actually aged more quickly when she sold the home than when she owned it. Depending on whether it was four or five years ago, she was either 93 or 94 when she still lived there... And, for example, I don't know if it was Monday or Tuesday, it was the day that she did the sheets. So she would take the sheets off her bed and she'd go to the beds upstairs and take all the sheets off, take them down in the basement, do the wash. She had an old wringer washer. She'd do all the wash. She'd dry it out and she'd put it all back on. That was Monday. Tuesday was something-else day. Wednesday was something-else day. One day was whatever, cleaning the kitchen or something like that. So she had these habits. And then every year in spring, she'd repaint the kitchen walls and the kitchen ceiling. Now she's 90-something now doing this. She had this tremendous routine.

Helena's rituals at home spread to her activities outside the home. In a systematic manner, she did activities in the city that pleased her and provided the structure that she wanted:

She would be done with her work for the day. And then her treat for herself would be to go outside, 'cause right on the corner she lived on there was a bus pick-up. So she would get on the bus and go to somewhere on Capital Drive, a little coffee shop or little restaurant. Stop for a cup of coffee and a piece of cake . . . And then she'd either come home or—she lived about three blocks away or two blocks away from the Kohl's food store. She'd come home if she had everything. If she didn't have everything, she'd take the bus to Kohl's and then she'd get food at Kohl's and walk home the last two blocks. So she had routines for everything. She fed the animals out back— the squirrels and the birds. She had a pear tree in the backyard. She canned the pears and gave a bunch away to her friends. She had certain decorations for certain holidays—especially Christmas was a biggie. And Easter was kind of a biggie. But her house was always clean and always in good order.

Expressing One's Self

Memories that suggest place as process also involve the dynamic of self-expression. We often personalize the physical environment with artifacts, pictures, furniture, and so on as part of making a place "our own." The apartments in a single building may be identical in design, but when lived in by different individuals, they reflect the people's different preferences for things and ways of arranging them and their lifestyles and personalities. One of the first things women do when they move into a new house is to hang pictures on the wall as a way of self-expression (Burnham, 1998). The act is the first step in making the home personal, transforming the faceless space into a personal place. Self-expression in an environment depends on, among other things, a perceived feeling of control and ownership.

Having the freedom to express ourselves in the spaces around us is key in making the space meaningful. Over time, the psychological investment in decorating, maintaining, and using a place can help develop a deep attachment. Residents' memories revealed that denial of self-expression and lack of a sense of belonging contributed to place experiences that were not remembered positively. Consider the case of Maria's perception of one of her childhood homes. Maria was living with her aunt, and because of various circumstances, she did not consider the home her own. This feeling was reflected in her daughter's recollection:

At the junior high time, when [Maria's] mother died, they moved and they lived in this flat above Gannon's Variety Store. And her aunt was Sis and her uncle was Joe Frank. And they owned and ran this store, this variety store. It was during the Depression . . . She never felt free to bring friends over because it wasn't really her own home, and there wasn't really much time, because of the help that she had to give there, to do much outside of the home. This was probably a time and place that my mother does not remember positively.

Often the house that provided the opportunity for self-expression was the one lived in after marriage. Before marriage, it was the "family home," the "parents' home," and although there was a feeling of belonging, there wasn't a feeling of ownership. Perhaps this need to express oneself is also tied with one's life stage. As individuals reach a certain age, they develop, their personalities mature, and the need or urge to express themselves increases. Marriage represented a chance to live in a place that provided scope for self-expression. In Maria's case, she finally found her "dream home," where she settled with her family. She expressed a sense that the house was "meant to be" for their family. One can sense a deep feeling of attachment on Maria's part for the house in later years. She often talked about the house to her adult children. I talked with her daughter, who recalled:

After [Mother and Father] had to keep moving from houses, they found a home. I guess they were ready to buy a home. It was on 25th Avenue, and that was in 1950 . . . It was roomy. It was two floors. And it had a nice yard. It had plenty of bedrooms because by that time there were five children, five of us. The location was excellent. All these things were there. Church. The Uptown. Any stores you wanted. Grocery store, drug store, all that. There was a school on each corner. There was a library right across the street. Post office a couple blocks away. A bank . . . [The house] was two blocks from the train station, and she had used that going back and forth to Milwaukee at different times. But that house was the answer to her prayers. That's how she talks about it. And the minute she saw it, she thought this was meant to be. So that was her dream house . . . She was there for 41 years—that was the time for her as a person when she came into her own, probably accomplished the most, was most involved and independent in her things, acquired positions in the

community and with her friends, plus how much her family means to her.
The house was probably the most important thing to her.

In Helena's case, her summer cottage seemed like more than a place for self-expression; it was a place where she felt rejuvenated and at peace with herself. The cottage was a retreat for her every summer, and she used to look forward to going back each June. There was sense of spiritual connectedness between Helena and her cottage—in her finding solace and mental peace. She talked about her cottage to her friend, who remembered:

Helena had a little lake cottage for many years that she sold about probably
12 years ago or 13 years ago. And that was a real big thing for her. That was her
own place . . . She not only talked about the lake and trees, but how she felt
that cottage was her source of strength and happiness. She told us how she
thought about the place when living in Milwaukee and how she planned on
doing new things once she would get back there. That was her pride and joy.

Choosing furniture, pictures, and the like is one form of self-expression. Another is adapting the place to suit personal needs and preferences. Being free to modify the physical surroundings is an important aspect of exercising territorial control and ownership. This may involve modification of the architectural environment or features of the space, such as painting walls, putting up wallpaper, renovating the kitchen, or building a closet.

These activities of physical modification symbolize one's territorial control over the home environment and reaffirm one's psychological connection with the home. In Maria's dream house, for example, everything was fine except that she wanted to change the siding and convert the front porch into a sunroom. Although she was not an expert in home renovation or repair, she had specific ideas about how some things could change in the house. She encouraged her husband to work on the house, and even after his death she continued to do some things on her own initiative. Maria's daughter described her involvement in the modification of her dream house:

It had siding that was sort of asphalt siding, and she never liked that siding.
And she always had hoped that they could re-side it. Although she asked my
father to get it done, Dad never got around to it. And after my father died,

she re-sided the house. It had a big porch in the front. And when we first moved there, that was open. Then after a while, maybe seven or eight years later, my father closed that in so that there were combination storm windows on it, and they had furniture out there. And my mother would go out there sometimes in the summer, in the evening after everything was done, and read out there, read the newspaper or whatever. So that was a pleasant place for her.

Raising a Family

Just as place as process is associated with expressing oneself, it is also intimately linked to the experience of raising a family. The majority of the women I interviewed were mothers and homemakers and spent a great deal of time taking care of their children. Having and raising children was one of the most significant activities of that cohort. From the moment of birth through the years of child rearing, the times of caring for children are significant events in one's life and are likely to be an important part of memories. These residents remembered home as the place for raising children and taking care of the family. Julia's daughter talked about the special home in her mother's life and how she felt that the home was something that was meant to be. Julia was a devoted and loving mother and wife; home was at the center of her world. But beyond the milieu where she expressed her love for her family, the house became part of her faith in a divinity. For Julia, that home seemed to have transcended the lived life to become something sacred in which she had deep belief. In her daughter's words:

She talks even in terms of divine providence with that home that was the house where she was supposed to have her family. She has very deep faith, and saying how she just felt that they were led there or it was what was meant to be . . . She remembers that home as she had lived there. One thing that I think is significant is, originally in Kenosha, the streets were named by names. Later they were all changed to numbers. And now very often when she talks about Kenosha, she'll say the named streets instead of the numbered streets.

In a related but somewhat different way, Brenda's love for her home represented her loyalty to and love for her husband. As her husband became sick, Brenda took care of him in the home for two years. She remembered her home to her daughter as a symbol of her commitment to and ties with her family. For Brenda, the home represented the process by which she took care of her husband and the ways in which she expressed her feelings for him. Her emotions about her family and home come through in her daughter's recounting:

My father had gotten sick in 1978. She took care of him in the home for two years. They got a hospital bed and put that in the dining room. She had visiting nurses come in. She was pretty well confined [so] that she could not just leave. And she was very active, so she'd always have to have people come and stay with him when she wanted to do things. But it very much limited her life, 'cause she loved to travel and was very involved in different things . . . The home kind of ties in with that. It's part of that—and she told me that this home was the representation of her love for family. It embodied the loyalty and the bond there.

Threading Memories from Generation to Generation

The attributes of place as process I've explored thus far center on the individual, even when the core lived experience involves others, such as children or a spouse. But the recollections shared by residents and their family members revealed that place as process also has an intergenerational dimension. Memories of one generation became part of those of the next, threaded across time and place. Although my interviews with the family members were focused on their loved one's past places, it wasn't uncommon for them to begin talking about the homes where they themselves grew up. Obviously, these homes are part of the memories of both generations. For the resident, typically the house was one of the places of adulthood, but for the daughter or son, it was the childhood home.

Maria's daughter remembered the closet that her father had built in their house and how she and her sisters made the cubbyhole their own little place. There was a sense of secrecy mixed with childlike joy about that place. This is her own memory of the house that held so many memories for her mother:

My father had finished off the bedroom with knotty pine and had made these closets and made a cubbyhole . . . and it was covered by a bookcase.

We thought it was so neat because it was like a spy movie or something. You could move that bookcase and then crawl in there, and that's where they stored all their pictures and different keepsakes and things like that. So we would sometimes love to go in there and just look through some of the things, when nobody was home or something. And then you could pull that bookcase back. My sisters and I thought that was our hideaway.

Memories of possessions as part of remembrance of places were discussed earlier. Possessions such as furniture help formulate a sense of self-identity, and remembering meaningful possessions can be considered remembering the self. Passing on special family artifacts as heirlooms to the next generation is not uncommon. Residents talked about their special furniture items and how these had been passed on to their offspring. There is a sense of self-continuity in this passing on of possessions, as if the things would symbolically carry on and maintain one's presence.

Attachment to Home

A final salient theme that emerged from the recollections of residents and their family members is that of attachment to home. For most of the residents interviewed, the home was the central setting of their life experiences. Significant life experiences and identity processes can create deep affective bonds between individuals and their homes. Home was at the core of life-course events for most of the women in this study who had been homemakers. In general, the social expectations and norms of the era in which they spent most of their adult years created a home-centered attitude and preference. Most family members recalled their loved ones' deep emotional associations with their homes. Like the themes of belonging to place, place anchors, and place as process, attachment to home has several facets. Each individual's experience of place was unique, shaped by the nature of the places he or she was involved with and by the individual's personality, needs, and personal interpretations, but the recollections shared certain threads of meaning: place as part of self, revisiting, longing, and divestment ritual. In some ways, place as a part of self subsumes the other shared meanings. It can be argued that both the urge for "revisiting" and "longing" evolve as place becomes part of self-identity. Similarly, psychological divestment as a process for consciously detaching oneself from a place reflects the integral role of that place in one's sense of self.

Place as Part of the Self

Homes emerged in these recollections as locations where personally meaningful life experiences took place. Through these subjective experiences, the homes had become strongly ingrained in the memories. Events, people, and places had become woven into the tapestries of residents' lives. As each one recollected her life, memories of special places came through as the context, ingredient, and anchors of events over the life course. In this process of acquiring deep personal meaning, homes became part of the residents' sense of self-identity.

Being attached to a home could mean material sacrifice. For Maria and her husband, there was a time when they had to choose between their home in Menomonie and the financial stability of the family. It was a home they had planned for and that Maria had grown to love over the years. To let go of the house and move out would have been to lose part of their self-identity. The home meant stability, love, and the sanctity of their family, and they decided to hold on to it. Maria's daughter, in her interview with me, mentioned that event in her mother's life a few times and added that Maria used to talk often about that difficult time in her life. Maria's story unfolded in her daughter's recollection:

In 1960, when my father was 60 years old, the company was going to move to Indiana. They were saying to him, you have to come along or something wouldn't come through with his pension or something . . . My parents really agonized over this. How could we leave this place? Leaving the city that they had both lived in just about all their lives? So they did make the decision, and I think they really leaned toward staying all along, but it was that they really had to consider giving up whatever that monetary thing was . . . They decided not to move because of not wanting to leave the city, not wanting to leave their home, that home, and wanting to keep the stability for us children. I think that time was very significant for my mother because she had told me this event several times. Although it was difficult for my parents to make the decision to stay back in Kenosha, my mother was very happy that they did.

Place as a part of self was illustrated in a literal and dramatic way by the story of Helena and her home. I interviewed Helena's friend (who had durable power of attorney) about places from her past. He talked about the story that Helena had shared with him numerous times. This was an incident in which her house was literally moved from one location to another, in accordance with her wishes. When the city asked Helena to move out of her house, which was to be torn down to make way for a new freeway, she could not accept the idea of being separated from it. For Helena, her home was an integral part of who she was, and to lose the home meant losing a part of herself. Perhaps Helena's case points out how the reality of moving out of one's home can reveal the emotional bonds one might have with a place. It is at the time of separation that we truly realize how much a person or place means to us. In Helena's story, the relationship between her home and herself was highlighted through a demonstration of her initiative. Her friend described this significant event in Helena's life:

> *It may have been '40s, but I think it was the '30s. And the house happened to be where the I-43 expressway was then. But the house got condemned because they literally lived where I-43 ended, right there. So Helena went in and talked to the county or whoever condemned it and made a deal where they paid them something for the land but she moved the house. And at that time, she moved it way west, to 27th and Capital. And that house stayed on 27th and Capital. In fact, it's still there. She was so attached to that home, and that home meant everything to her.*

At the other end of spectrum was Mary, who never wanted to own a home and indeed seems to have shied away from developing an attachment with home. Although her husband could afford to buy a home, they always chose to rent. This seemed strange to her son, who decided that not owning a home was Mary's way of expressing a different psychological reality. For example, there are people who avoid getting into a personal relationship for fear of losing that person. In so doing these individuals recognize their own fears and emotions and take steps to provide a psychological safeguard of sorts. Mary's son saw a similar motivation behind his mother's never wanting to buy a home in all her adult years:

Mother did not ever want to buy a home. That was something strange . . . She was such a good homemaker and took pride in doing things around the home, but did not want to buy a home. My father wanted to buy one and was financially very much able to do so, but did not buy because of her. Could be because she did not want permanent attachment. I think that was her way of coping with the possibility of losing something that did not happen anyway.

Attachment to one's home was also expressed in decisions to hold on to a place that could provide a sense of stability. For some, like Maria, frequent moving could affect relationships with these aspects of place, as if there wasn't enough time to settle down and nourish and maintain them. Having had that experience in childhood, Maria developed a desire for stability for her own children. Maria shared her values with her daughter. In her daughter's words:

One of the things, my mother says this often—as far as not having to move anymore—she'll often say, because her mother died so young and then her father, she'll say, "I always prayed that I would live long enough to raise my children." And then we'll say, "Yeah," and not only that, but we did have such stability that I say, for myself, that all but two years of my whole childhood were in that one home. And I think that was very important to her because of relating it to her mother.

Expression of love for a place can take various forms and shapes. For Maria and her husband, it meant giving up financial security; for Helena, it meant taking the home along with her as she moved. Michael expressed emotion for his home in a more poignant and touching way. Michael's attachment to his home was apparent through his talking about the home with the staff in his initial years in the nursing home. After a few years, his cognitive status declined, and he did not talk about the home as he had before. However, one incident graphically depicts his attachment to his home. His brother narrated:

I think the first home Mike purchased on Story Parkway in Milwaukee was the first place he really enjoyed and was happy with . . . He misses his present home very, very much and talked about it all the time to the staff. When June and I visited him shortly after he was admitted to the present Sunrise

Nursing Home, we took him back to his house for a weekend. When we arrived at his present home in Brookfield, he got down on his hands and knees and kissed the floor—very moving and sad gesture. I know he is deeply pained that he is not living out his final years in his home that he loves so much.

Revisiting a Place

Just as personally meaningful places were significant in respondents' recollections, so was a desire to revisit those places. Recollection of place experiences can serve as a surrogate for physical visits to those places. However, in the event of an actual visit to a personally meaningful place from the past, the physical immediacy of the place can provide strong cues for recollection. Linda's niece talked about how her aunt liked revisiting her childhood home when she had an opportunity. Linda had dementia and was living in Crescent Nursing Home. Her only relative was her niece, who lived in a different state. Although Linda didn't share much about her home-related feelings with her niece, she always wanted to take a ride by her old home when her niece was visiting her. Her niece described her aunt's wishes:

I remember the house very well. It was a one-story house that she lived in with her mother, father, and brother. She and her brother were twins. He passed away 8/20/92. The house had a small front yard with a double swing in it. She definitely missed her childhood home. When I lived in Milwaukee, she always wanted to go for a ride past that house.

In Julia's case, an important part of her childhood revolved around her times at her grandparents' farm in Nebraska. As an adult, she carried fond memories of her experiences there and took a trip with her family to revisit the place. The revisiting was a special event for Julia, and she talked about it in detail to her daughter. At the time of this study, Julia had dementia and was living in a nursing home. Her cognitive decline had been rapid, and she did not communicate much with her daughter. Julia's daughter felt that her mother still had a sense of attachment to her grandparents' farm and that maybe she would take her there once again. She said:

Years and years later, when my parents were well into their retirement, they took a trip back there and visited that home. And the fact that they looked for that home, I would say, probably means that it was quite special to her. She spent a lot of childhood days there . . . They found the home. They went into it. The people that lived there let them come in. I do remember that she told me about their visit there, that they went up the stairs and she said, "I remember as a little girl there was always a bookshelf on this landing." You know, the stairs would go up so much, and then there'd be a landing, and then there'd be more stairs up to the top. And on that landing there was a bookshelf with a lot of books in it. And in the summer, that's how she spent some of her time, sitting there reading those books. And so, when she went back then, as an older [person] (I would say she was probably in her 70s at that time that she went back), she would have sworn that same bookshelf with the same books was still there. She said, "I couldn't believe it. It just looked exactly the same," the way she remembered it. So that was significant, I think.

Revisiting a place could be part of maintaining a family's history. One of Brenda's homes was a farm in New York, where her daughter spent some of her childhood as well. When I talked with Brenda's daughter, she recalled the farm from her own childhood. She also remembered the time that she took her own family, including her grandchildren, to visit that childhood home. For Brenda's daughter, the farm represented part of her own childhood as well as her parents' place. Perhaps that visit to the farm represented both a desire to visit a special place from her own past and an opportunity to pass on the memories of that farm to future generations. Visits to the parental home could provide and reinforce a sense of belonging and continuity for herself and her family. The farm was a physical manifestation of family lineage that had spanned more than four generations. Brenda's daughter remembered the home from her early years as well as from the time of that visit in later years:

This farm was in New York, but it was on the edge of the Vermont state line. And there were a lot of skiers in the area, and my mother took in people who were looking for a place to stay, who came to ski, and she took in hunters. There was one end of the house we didn't use. And it was not in use because they slept upstairs over the main portion of the house. Someone had built a wing with rooms. We went back with our grandchildren; we wanted to show them our own neighborhood where we grew up.

Longing

Closely related to the attachment to home as a sense of place that is a part of the self is the longing for that special place. The word *longing* suggests a yearning for something that is a long way off, something that we belong to and that belongs to us. The longing for home is a universal form of longing that is expressed in the English language as *homesickness*. But the word *homesickness* has a connotation of an isolated condition that seems temporally bounded. If I am homesick, I will feel better when I get home. The word *longing* implies a broader yearning for a thing, person, or place that may transcend temporal boundaries and can survive for an extended period of time. Some of the residents' life stories conveyed a sense of longing for emotionally significant places—a longing that persisted if the revisit or visit never happened. In such cases, the longing did not die away, but lingered, like a low flame. Consider Helena's longing to go back to Germany, the land of her birth. She came to the United States in childhood and had never had a chance to revisit her birthplace. The trip was planned but not taken. Her friend described Helena's longing for her birthplace:

> *Shortly after moving to the nursing home, she made arrangements to tour Germany. This was something she had wanted to do for most of her life. She told me that she would like to visit the town and home where she was growing up a child. But my father, Paul, passed away on the day she would have departed. She elected to postpone the tour to a later date, and never got around to it again.*

Divestment Ritual

Strong emotional attachment to place also means that we need to find ways to separate ourselves emotionally from places when we must move away from them physically. The need can be especially acute when the move is not toward some desired goal but is unwelcome. Rituals of divestment emerged as a common thread in the interviews.

People typically move from a place to another place with a purpose: moving to a more desirable home, moving to take a job, moving for the sake of education. Such purposes make the move bearable; one has something to look forward to. However, when health fails, children move out, or friends and neighbors pass away, elderly people may move to a nursing home, and such a move is the formal beginning of the end for the elderly individual. This is a rite of passage no one wishes to face. Leaving one's home can be a deeply emotional experience. How do people let go of home and the lives they have lived?

In some residents' recollections, one coping mechanism was a ritual of saying goodbye to the home. As in a divestment ritual, the individuals did things such as going back to the empty house for one last time, taking photographs of the house, or talking about the home after the move. For Helena, moving out of her home, though she eventually came to terms with it, was psychologically difficult. As a ritual of divesting herself of her attachment to the home, she wanted to spend one last night there. For her, a night's stay was a way of closing a chapter in her life, and by doing that, she symbolically detached herself from her home. Helena's moving-out ritual was narrated by her friend as follows:

> We were getting ready for the moving date and little by little moving things over that we thought she'd like. And then the day of the move. So we moved her over, got her bed set up, got all the furniture in she was gonna take. We brought too much stuff, but we brought what she wanted and had her room set up. And she said, "Okay, let's go home now." And we said, "No, you can't go home." She said, "I want to go home." We hadn't put the house up for sale yet 'cause I wanted her to be able to move out without putting her under any pressure . . . We finally made an agreement with her . . . where she would go to her house for one more day, or one more night in it. So she went back to her house, stayed in her house one more night. We figured the next day, when my wife [went] to pick her up, that she was gonna fight tooth and nail. Nope, she was fine. They had a nice breakfast. And my wife dropped her off in her new home, and she was fine. She was all done.

Memories such as those presented above and other home-related information from residents, their family members, or their close friends can form the basis for "home stories"—home-related biographical sketches of residents in nursing homes and dementia care units. Home stories can help the staff see residents as individuals who worked, raised families, were part of communities, and lived rich lives before they moved out of their homes and into the nursing home. Home stories can also be the basis for guided reminiscence conversations with residents. Used alone or with photographs of residents' former homes and other significant places from their past, home stories can help residents reconnect with a sense of self.

CHAPTER FOUR

"That Is My Home"

Home Stories and Guided Conversations

> I looked up the steep hill and saw the backyard that nurtured
> me and I remembered the swamp where little peepers
> serenaded spring, while freight trains passed slowly. I yearn
> to walk up the steep hills and wander through the backyard
> full of memories lost so long ago. Would the present
> occupants understand if I told them I wanted one last look at
> a link of my life before I died of Alzheimer's?
>
> —*Thomas DeBaggio,* When It Gets Dark *(2003)*

As Tom DeBaggio started to write about his life after being diagnosed with Alzheimer disease, he frequently mentioned his home and neighborhood. His vivid recollection of his home and what it meant to him speaks powerfully about the place of home in our lives. Often we remember and share our lives in the form of stories or narratives.

There are three primary approaches to viewing the nature of life narratives. The first approach holds that a narrative of life experiences is a means of understanding the historical facts of an individual's life. In this approach, communicated life experience is seen as an objective representation of events and experiences (Polkinghorne, 1988). The second approach emphasizes the subjective aspects of life stories. Instead of focusing on life narratives as objective accounts of experience, this view emphasizes the individual's perceptions, values, definitions of situations, and personal goals. A third approach views life narratives as social constructions, as created, shaped, and sustained by the social and cultural contexts of the individuals (Gubrium, 1993). Individual subjectivity cannot be separated from the social structure within which it is embedded. Thus, this third approach sees an individual's memories of past places recounted in place stories as subjective and influenced by the sociological context in which the individual exists.

Narrative communication is an attempt to distill the passions, desires, ideas, pain, joy, and laughter of human experience into some meaningful arrangement of words. As a bird in a cage can spread its wings but cannot fly, so the essence of experience is caged by words. It is the listener/reader's *interpretation* of the narrative that gives meaning, or rather reassigns meaning, to someone else's life experience. We share our life experiences primarily through words. We rely on narratives in telling our stories and in understanding and drawing meaning from others' stories. Understanding experience through narrative contextualizes the events and stories related in the personal and social realities of places, events, and other individuals.

In retelling "home stories" passed on to them by their parents or other family members, individuals may add their subjective interpretations. This dynamic social aspect of the recollections of events, perceptions, and emotions signifies the social construction of home stories. Thus, home stories not only reflect the past as transmitted by a loved one with dementia but also may include stories passed on by a parent, elder sibling, close relative, or family friend. The home stories reproduced here summarize the focused biographies of residents whom we met in the previous chapter through the narratives of their family members or friends. The stories are presented in the format in which the data were collected, to illustrate the narrative nature of the original data. These five stories of place illustrate the diversity and richness of the residents' life experiences. The diversity is reflected in various features, such as residents' childhood places (e.g., farm, small city, large city) and frequency of moves.

Helena (as related by her friend Andrew)
Moving to the United States

Helena was born in 1898 and raised in Germany. Her family had a tavern, with Dad taking care of the bar business and Mom making the food. As a child, she was expected to help her mother with the food preparation as best she could. In the 1920s, at the age of 22, she moved from Germany to the United States. She and her husband had saved enough money to take the trip. The voyage over set her up with a good attitude on arriving in the United States—Helena learned hairdressing in Germany and became rather good at it. Although she suffered from motion sickness on the ship that forced her to stay in bed for two or three days, all of the affluent women on the ship wanted her to do their hair. By the time the ship arrived in New York, she earned a $20 gold piece. At that time that was enough money to make a down payment on a house. But the gold piece was dated 1898, the year she was born. Helena took this as a sign of good luck and kept the gold piece her entire life.

Working

Helena got a job at Schuster's [a department store] as a hairdresser in the 1930s, when it was called Gimbel-Schuster's. The Depression was hard on Helena and her husband. Money was tight—so tight that they had to give up their first home. He was a designer for A. O. Smith [a corporation that manufactures water heaters] but was laid off during the hard times. Helena stayed with Gimbel-Schuster's while her husband was out of work into the 1940s. By the time her husband had gotten his job back, they were renting the upstairs of their second house to roomers to pay the mortgage. The roomers had helped them immensely to carry on through the Depression. Once the couple was back on their feet, Helena's job was to take care of the house and the roomers.

The Dream House

Helena's dream house was in Milwaukee where I-43 ends. Her husband had the house built in the '30s. In the '40s, the house was condemned because they literally lived where I-43 was to end. When she heard that she had to give up her home, Helena was stricken. She was attached to that home, and it meant everything to her. So she marched in and talked to the county officials, making a deal with them that they would pay her for the land and pay to have the house moved to another location.

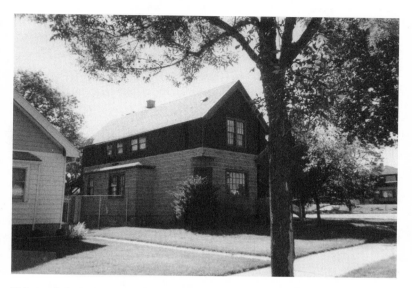

Helena's home, which was literally moved from its original location to another neighborhood in the same city at Helena's request. The city was planning to tear the house down because of freeway construction.

Helena chose a location that was at that time far west at 27th and Capital, and her house was moved to that spot.

The house was exactly what she wanted. There was one bedroom on the first floor, and the second floor had five small bedrooms. During the Depression, when her husband lost his job, Helena had started renting the rooms out to make ends meet. Her tenants were mostly young men just arrived from Germany, barely able to speak English. They lived upstairs and paid her by the week. She would take them under her wing and take care of them. They had dozens of people live with them throughout the years, and some of them became lifelong friends. One man in particular, Jimmy, lived with them for more than 20 years. He kept contact with her for a long time.

After her husband died, Helena used the money from the tenants to sustain her lifestyle; she also enjoyed the company. She continued to live in the house until 1993, when she decided to move. Although she had great neighbors who were nice to her and watched out for her, she knew the house was getting to be too much for her. In 1993, she moved out of the house and into Milwaukee Catholic Home. The first night in the nursing home was difficult for her. So she moved back to her home and spent one last night in the house that held all her memories. The next day she moved everything she wanted to take with her into her new apartment, and after that she never looked back. She was attached to that home; it meant everything to her. But as much as the house meant to her, once she moved out, she didn't ever talk about it.

Taking Care of the House

Helena was particular about the upkeep of her house. She had an everything-in-order mentality that was expressed in her meticulous housekeeping. Her routine was strict. Some housekeeping task was scheduled for each day. On Monday, it was changing the sheets. She would take the sheets off her bed, take them down to the basement, and do the wash in her old wringer washer. When she was finished, she would hang them to dry, and when they were dry, she'd remake all the beds. Tuesday was tidying-up-the-kitchen day. And so forth. On some days, once she was done with the housework, she would go out and treat herself. Right on the corner of her street there was a bus stop. So she would get on the bus and go to a little coffee shop or restaurant. She would have a cup of coffee and a piece of cake. And then she would either go home or go to the Kohl's food store about three blocks away from her home. She would buy something from the store and walk home.

Every year in spring, she would repaint the kitchen walls and ceiling. Taking care of the outside of her house was just as important to her as keeping up the inside. She fed the animals out back—the squirrels and the birds. She had a pear tree in the backyard. Every year she used to can pears and give them away to her friends. She made sure every holiday was festively decorated for, especially Christmas and Easter. She continued this routine into her 90s, quitting only when she moved out of the house.

Home away from Home

Helena had a little lake cottage for many years on Lake Winnebago. The cottage was a summer place where she and her husband used to

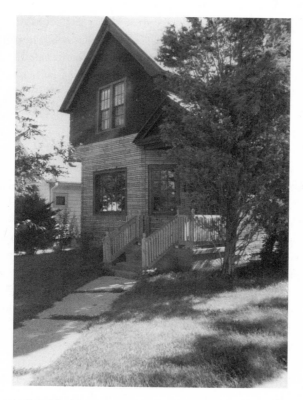

Helena liked to watch the seasons through the living
room's large windows

spend time. At the end of each summer, they closed it up. When they
came back the following year, she would always do a lot of cleaning in the
first few days. In the early days when she was doing work inside, her
husband would be working outside. But after he died, she did all the work
inside and outside. It was a small, clean cottage. There were two small
bedrooms, a small living room, a bathroom, and a kitchen. Helena liked
the cozy atmosphere of the cottage. The decorating style in the cottage was
similar to that of her home, representing the dominant styles of the 1940s
and '50s. The tables had metal legs; the chairs had tubular steel frames to
which cushions were attached. It wasn't anything fancy, but it was clean,
and that's the way she liked to keep it. There was a chair in her living room

that she really liked. It was an easy chair where she could sit and use a remote control to switch the TV on and change channels. She used to stay up until midnight or one o'clock, sitting in that chair, watching TV, reading, or knitting.

The Flood

Not long after Helena's husband died, there was a horrible rain. There were farmers' fields all around the lake, and the cottage was at the bottom of the hill, pretty close to the water. A little creek ran beside her cottage. The creek held the runoff from those farmers' fields. The fields flooded, and the water from the creek rushed through and knocked out the foundation of the cottage. Her boat was pushed out into the lake. Her chairs were washed away, and all her paintings were knocked over. Helena was upset. It was one of the worst things in the world for her, and she needed help. Her nephew came to look and said something like, "Oh, this place is worthless now. It's gonna need to be rebuilt. And you can't do any of this. Why don't you sell it to me for $5?" Helena did sell it off for $5, but since then she hasn't ever wanted to have anything to do with her nephew.

Sheila (as related by her nephew Michael)
Childhood Years on a Farm

Sheila was born in March 1901 on a farm in upper Michigan. Her birth name was Radtke. Her parents had emigrated from Germany in the 1880s. Sheila was a farm girl—born and raised on the family farm. In those days farming was not a money-making activity; it was survival for the family. So the entire family labored on the farm. Sheila and her siblings worked hard every day of the year.

Her childhood home was a single-family three-bedroom wood-frame structure, without running water or electricity. The porch had a swing, which was a popular place to sit in summer. Sheila used to love swinging there at the end of the day. There was also a one-room detached house, which was kept for visitors. Toilet facilities were outdoor privies; water was carried in from a well. Candles and lanterns provided light. Simple things, such as soap, were homemade, and no basic necessities were

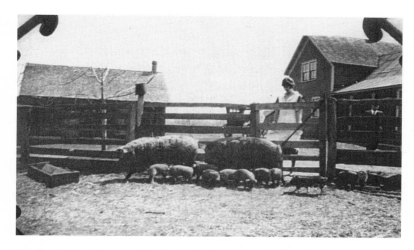

The family farm in upper Michigan where Sheila was born and where she grew up. The building on the right was the house where she lived. The structure on the left was a machine shed.

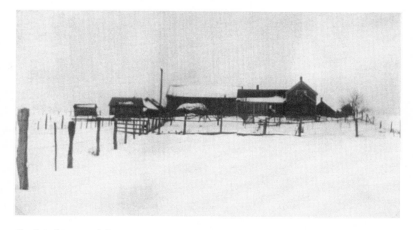

Sheila's farmstead during winter, as seen from the north. The barn and granary were to the left of the house.

bought from the store. She enjoyed her years on the farm. She was especially fond of the pigs and mentioned having a pet pig. Living on the farm
allowed her maximum time to explore nature and her world, to dream,
invent activities, and make use of the available materials and resources to
create her own fun.

Besides working in the farm, Sheila's activities included learning to
dance, playing games such as crack-the-whip, sledding and ice skating
during the winter when conditions allowed, knitting and tatting, and
corn-husking parties. There wasn't much time for just plain old fun. Most
of the activities were work/survival related. In other words, people had to
make work into fun for obvious reasons. She often said, "We had to make
our own fun." Perhaps one of the reasons this was possible was the fact
that her relatives and neighbors were all in the same social and economic
situation. They had to help each other, and they turned that help into
social, fun activities.

The Cottage by the River Escanaba

Sheila's father built a cottage by the River Escanaba, which was a tribu-
tary of the Fox River. She helped her father saw the logs into lumber for
the cottage. She loved fishing and spent a lot of time at the cottage during
summers with her father and half-sister Louise. Her father and she liked
fishing so much that they decided to finish the side of the cottage with
fish-scale-like siding. A few years after her father's death, the family decided to sell the cottage. Sheila was reluctant to let the cottage go. After the
cottage was sold, she went back and made friends with the new owner.
She told her nephew in later years that the cottage was a tie to her father, to
whom she had been attached. Returning to that cottage and the river was
like being close to her father.

Milwaukee as Home

When Sheila moved to Milwaukee with her husband, she loved the city.
The places she lived were all near the central city, within walking distance
of downtown. From the isolation of childhood, she seemed to have gravi-
tated to the hustle of the central city. She was proud to be of German

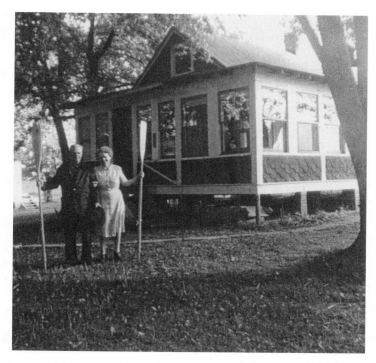

Sheila and her husband, John, in front of the cottage by the River Escanaba. Her family did not own the house at the time this picture was taken, but she used to visit the place occasionally in memory of her father.

origin, and Milwaukee, at that time, was a predominantly German city. She spoke the language and had been raised surrounded by German culture. The social and cultural contexts of Milwaukee seemed to naturally draw her. She spent her entire adult life in that city.

The first apartment she lived in was on 18th Street. It was on the second floor and had one bedroom, living and dining in one space, and a bathroom. There were two things that she liked about the apartment. The living room had a window facing east, and she just loved the morning sunlight in summer. She used to sit in her rocking chair, looking out the window, the sun shining on her feet, sipping the day's first cup of coffee. Although she would have preferred a little more space in the apartment, she was happy with it, especially because it had the east window. Also, Sheila liked the activity on 18th Street. It made her feel that she was not alone. Although later on she lived in larger apartments on Wells Street, she never liked those places as much as she had her first apartment in Milwaukee.

Travel

Sheila and husband, John, traveled extensively throughout the United States and Canada after he retired. She maintained a scrapbook detailing the things they saw and the places they visited. As much as she liked traveling to other places, she always wanted to visit Germany. Shortly after moving to the nursing home, she made arrangements to tour Germany. This was something she had wanted to do for most of her life. But her brother Paul passed away on the day she would have departed, and she decided to postpone the tour to a later date. She has never gotten around to it again.

Maria (as related by her daughter Rebecca)
The House in Menomonie

Maria was born in summer of 1914 in Menomonie, Wisconsin. Her father was a caretaker for the fairgrounds, and her family lived in a house on the fairgrounds. There was a front porch on the house and steps where she often sat. The house had a living and dining room, a kitchen, and a bedroom downstairs. There were two bedrooms upstairs. Maria was fascinated by the paint on the window frame in the room where she and her sister used to sleep. The paint of the window frame was peeling off, and Maria used to eat pieces of the old paint. She used to spend hours observing the cracks in old white paint and kept track of how the paint was gradually coming off the window frame. In fact, once she wrote an essay for her school assignment on how the paint had its own life and how it was growing old. Maria also liked the animals around the fairgrounds. Her father took care of the horses and other animals. Maria loved the chickens and a dog. She also loved wildlife, especially deer.

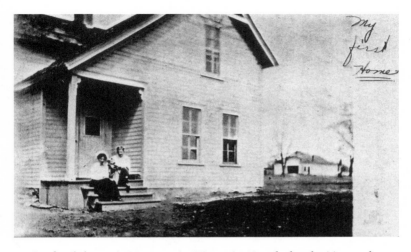

Maria's family home, in Menomonie, Wisconsin. Note the handwriting on the right side, "My first home," written by Maria before she was diagnosed with Alzheimer disease.

Eau Claire, Wisconsin

When Maria was about seven or eight, her family moved to Kenosha, where she went to elementary school. The week before her junior high school graduation, her mother died. After that, her aunt in Eau Claire, Wisconsin, wanted Maria and her brother to come there to go to school. They lived in a flat above Frank's Variety Store, on Main Street. Her aunt Sis and uncle Joe Frank owned and ran the variety store. It was during the Depression. Maria was not quite comfortable with the home in Eau Claire. Although she liked the Main Street neighborhood, she couldn't feel totally at home there, primarily because she knew it wasn't their place.

After living in Eau Claire for three years, when she was in high school, Maria and her brother moved back to Racine. They had relatives in Racine with whom she was close. Maria and her brother rented an apartment across the street from her aunt Melia's. She liked the apartment and talked about it often. She talked about furnishing the place. They bought a few pieces of furniture, like a couch, a desk, and a lamp, from rummage sales. There was a bookcase that she liked. Maria liked to read and was a

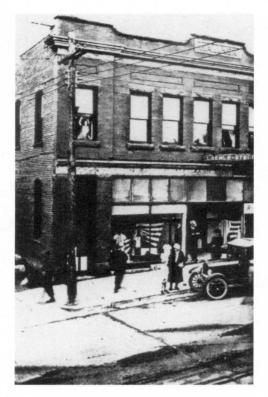

Uncle Joe's apartment and store, in Eau Claire,
Wisconsin, where Maria and her brother stayed for
some time

member of a Book of the Month Club. Once she bought a set of encyclopedias, and a bookcase came with it for free. She was fond of it and carried it
with her to different homes over the years. They used to live in the upper
flat of the house. She talked about the dark hardwood floor; she liked the
feel of that floor and usually walked barefoot in the house.

The Dream House

Maria's dream house was on 27th Avenue in Racine. She moved to that
house with her husband in 1951. The uptown location was excellent. A

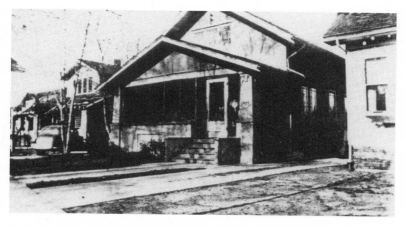

Maria's family home, in Racine, Wisconsin. Maria lived with her brother in the upper flat.

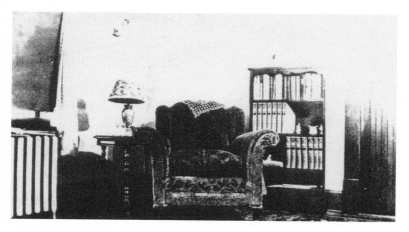

Maria's bookcase. She was very fond of the bookcase, which came with a set of encyclopedias she had purchased.

church, grocery store, and a drugstore were close. There was a school on the corner, a library right across the street, a post office a couple of blocks away, and a bank two blocks from the train station. The house was the answer to her prayers. That's how she talked about it. The minute she saw it, she knew this was meant to be. It had a nice yard. Her husband had

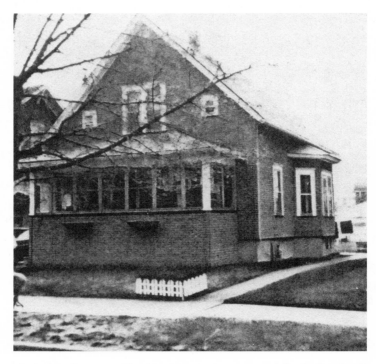

The house where Maria lived for more than 41 years with her husband and children

fixed it up—made changes that accommodated the family. Maria's five children were born there, and they grew up there. That house was home to Maria for more than 41 years.

The house had two stories. Initially, it had asphalt siding, which Maria never liked. She always had hoped that they could re-side it. After her husband died, she re-sided the house. When they first moved there, the house had an open front porch. Then, after seven or eight years, her husband closed it in so that there were combination storm windows on it. Maria would go out there sometimes in the summer, in the evenings after everything was done, and sit in a wicker chair and read. On the first floor there were two rooms—the living room and dining room—and there was an archway between them. There was a big bay window in the front that looked out onto the porch. Right off the living room there was a room where her brother lived for a few years. Later on it was made into the children's playroom. Her husband had his desk in there, and she had her sewing machine. She spent a lot of time in there sewing.

Although the kitchen was small, Maria liked it because of the cupboards. There was a big walk-in pantry that she loved. The kitchen table took up the middle of the kitchen. There was a bathroom off the kitchen, which she didn't like. Right before the pantry there were the stairs to the basement. She washed the clothes for a family of seven in the basement where the washer was located, and then she hung the clothes outside on the clothesline. She spent a lot of time in the basement.

The stairway had a door at the top so that the second floor could be closed off. There was a little hall at the top of the stairs, and to the right was her bedroom. Maria liked the big walk-in closet with her bedroom. Straight in front of the head of the stairs was the girls' room. There were four girls, so that was a longer bedroom. Her husband had finished the room in knotty pine and made the closets and a cubby-hole that was covered with a bookcase. The children thought it was like something from a spy movie. They could move the bookcase and crawl in there. That's where they stored all their pictures and different keepsakes. Left down the hall was the boy's room, which was much smaller than the others.

The yard was beautiful. There were two apple trees on one side, and the other side was set up for the kids' play area. Her husband had built a swing set for the children. There was a patch of dirt where the kids spent a lot of time playing. The rest of the yard was grass, and the children weren't supposed to wreck it. There were vegetables and flowers all along the sides of the yard and along the sides of and in front of the house.

The neighborhood was in the heart of the city. However, it was a residential area and was safe. It was the kind of place where people didn't have to lock their doors. There were all kinds of neighbors. There was a kind older couple and a German lady who became a good friend of Maria's. It was a pleasant neighborhood, and Maria wanted nothing else.

Staying Put

Maria's husband, Sam, worked at the SleepWell Mattress Company for 42 years. In 1960, when he was 60 years old, the company was preparing to move to Indiana. They wanted Sam to go along or else they wouldn't provide his pension. But how could he and Maria leave their home? She loved the house, the neighborhood, and the neighbors. So they made the decision to stay. He found a job as a custodian at a boarding school in Racine. In 1978, Sam got sick. Maria took care of him in their home for two years. They got a hospital bed and put it in the dining room. Although she was active socially, she cut down on her commitments to take care of her husband. One of their daughters wanted the hospital bed to be in the playroom so that Sam wouldn't be out in the open. But Maria insisted that Sam be out in the flow of their life where he could look out the windows and see if people were walking by on the street. He would be right in the midst of people coming in. She had talked about divine providence in terms of the family's staying in the house. She had deep faith and she felt that it was meant to be. The home embodied the love, the loyalty, and the bond between Maria and her husband.

Travel

In 1960, the couple bought their first car. Every summer, and sometimes in between, they would go to see the older girls, who were in Superior, Wisconsin. They would make it a week's vacation—go out to see them and then go to Eau Claire and Menomonie. They'd see the Franks in Eau Claire and the home on the fairgrounds of Menomonie. Maria enjoyed those trips very much. They went to a lot of different state campgrounds. After her husband died, Maria began taking each of the kids on a trip. Every summer she'd take a different one of the children, and he or she could pick where to go. She still remembers those trips and the car that they drove. She loved camping and visiting historical old houses. Even now, when she goes out with her daughter driving somewhere, she'll always point out an old house when she sees one.

Julia (as related by her daughter Maggie)
Memorable Places in Her Childhood Years

Julia was born on April 5, 1911, in Milwaukee, Wisconsin. Her family soon moved to New London, Wisconsin, where her father took a teaching

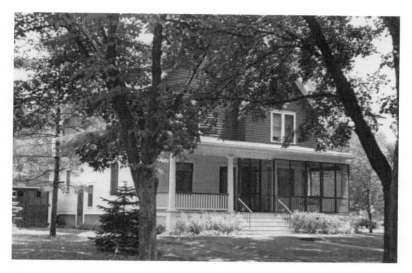

Julia's childhood home, in New London, Wisconsin

job. The first home she would remember was the house in New London on 14th Street. That was her home until 1932, when she got married. She has warm memories of that home, especially of her father's study. Her father was a professor, and he spent a lot of time in his study. Julia was fond of her dad and spent a lot of time in his study with him. The walls of the study were lined with books. She grew up to be an avid reader and book collector.

Julia's bedroom was upstairs. Her best friend, Betty, lived next door, and the houses were fairly close to each other. In fact, their bedroom windows faced each other. Sometimes they put up little pulleys, stretched string between two windows, and passed messages back and forth. She also talked about the large porch and the front yard. She and her friends played in the yard and on the porch in summer. Once they built a cardboard house on the porch and gave it the name "porch house." The "porch house" had a door and a window. To Julia, the porch was so large that it seemed as if their actual house could fit onto it.

Summers in Springfield, Nebraska

In the summers, Julia's family took a lot of trips to her father's family home in Springfield, Nebraska. Her grandfather and grandmother lived on a farm there. Because her father was a professor, he had the summers free. So they would pack up their whole family for the summer and basically live in Nebraska. Julia used to help her father on the farm. She loved those summers on the farm. The heat was memorable. There was an icehouse, where she would go whenever there was an opportunity. She liked the open fields and loved running as fast as she could. The farmhouse where her grandparents lived was a two-story structure with a bookcase landing. The house had a long porch that wrapped around the front and sides, where Julia and her cousins played hide and seek. One time while she was on the farm, there was a big lightning storm. She remembers being in bed that night and watching the lightning through the window. In her imagination, the lightning was like a raging horse made of fire playing with wind and water.

Grandma's Place and Knitting

Julia also loved to visit her grandma and grandpa, who owned a general store in Milwaukee. They lived in a flat above the store. When she visited them in Milwaukee, Julia liked to walk along the street and see different things in the shop windows. There was one shop named Little Things and More in that neighborhood. In its window was a miniature town complete with a school, office, church, stores, and railway station. In fact, that shop was one of the main attractions when she visited Grandma's place in Milwaukee. The other attraction was Grandma herself. Julia always felt she was a favorite of Grandma. Grandma taught her how to knit when she was five years old. And she's proud that she learned to knit so young. Some of her cousins couldn't catch on as she did, and she's proud of that. Braided rugs were another interest of hers. She liked to go to Grandma's house because she knew that Grandma would sit down with her and teach her how to make things.

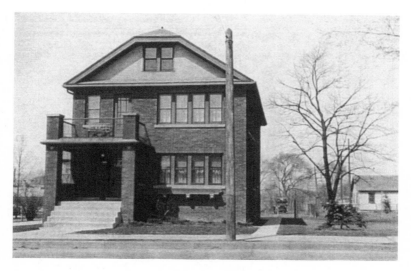

The house where Julia and her husband lived in the upper flat

The Flat in Waukesha, Wisconsin

At the age of 20, Julia married Frank, and they moved to a flat in Waukesha, Wisconsin. At first she did not like life in the city and went back to visit her parents in New London every month. However, after their first son was born she settled in and adjusted well to that flat and life in the city. Julia was an excellent homemaker, and besides keeping up with regular housekeeping tasks, she made some small-scale renovations in the flat. She changed the wallpaper in the living room and painted the kitchen cupboards. She also did a lot of cooking in those years. The kitchen in that flat was nice, with a large window overlooking the park. The view in autumn was breathtaking. After living there nine years, in 1941 they moved to a house on 42nd Street in Pewaukee.

Pewaukee, Wisconsin

Julia was always a nature lover. She liked to do things outdoors. The house they moved to in Wauwatosa had a large front yard with two apple trees. She started to garden and began to spend time in the yard every day

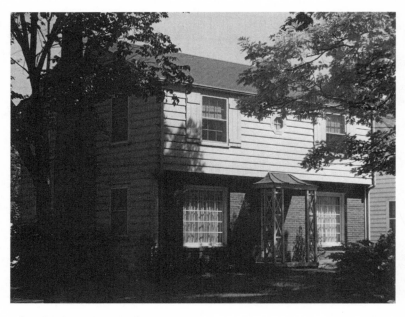

Julia's first home in Pewaukee, Wisconsin

in the spring and summer. There was a nearby park, where she and one of her neighbors went walking often. She liked the house except for one thing: she wished for a porch like the one she had at the house in New London. In fact, Julia planned to save money to build a porch someday. Her wish remained just a wish, as they moved to Chicago a few years later and sold the house.

Chicago . . . and California

By 1955, Julia's husband had established himself in business, and they moved to a suburb of Chicago called Eastport. She always took her husband to the train station, where he caught the train into downtown Chicago, the Loop, to work. She remembers taking him to the train station every day. She enjoyed driving back to her home through their quiet, peaceful neighborhood.

In 1960 Frank took a job with a company in California. Julia did not have a pleasant time in California. She felt that the neighborhood houses

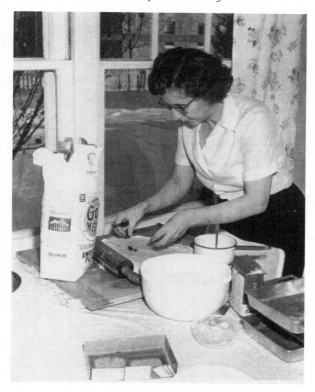

Julia working in her kitchen

were farther apart in California than they were in Wisconsin. And the owners did not build them, as had been the case in Wisconsin. She didn't feel quite secure because the houses did not have basements, and they didn't have the look of "Midwest solidity." Although it was a glamorous house in California with palm trees on the street and sunshine, she didn't feel at home. They did not stay there long but moved back to Wisconsin after two years.

Homecoming

They moved back to Pewaukee, where they had lived before. When they moved back, they lived in an apartment for a little while because Frank was building their dream home. It was her husband's dream home,

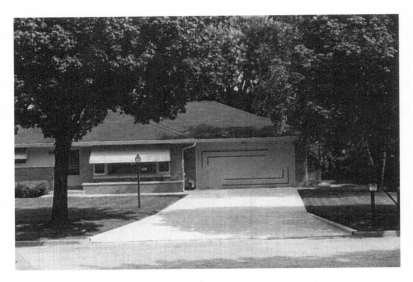

Julia's second Pewaukee home

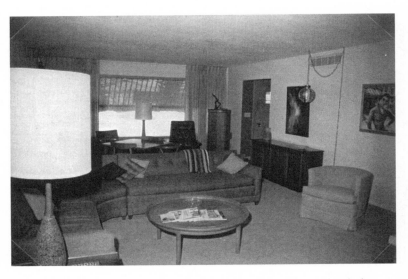

Julia was a good homemaker. This picture of her living room was taken by her husband.

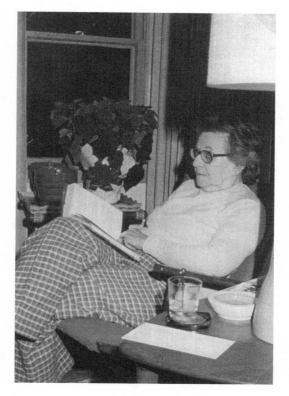

Julia's favorite spot in her home. She liked the view of
the garden through the window.

but it became a beloved home of Julia's as well. It was a lovely home on
Terrace Street. She was comfortable in that home. It was not glamorous, it
was modest, but she felt secure because it was in a familiar neighborhood.
It wasn't far from 42nd Street, where they had lived before, and she had
fond memories of the area.

Julia liked to take walks through the wooded neighborhood and the
homes that were close to each other. Her favorite place in their house in
Pewaukee was a comfortable chair in the living room. She used to sit there
every afternoon and either knit or read.

Before the Move to a Nursing Home

In the mid-1990s Julia's husband, Frank, became too ill to stay at home. After he was moved into a nursing home, Julia's health started to fail, and she was not able to keep up with the home. Maggie was afraid to leave her mother alone. The home in Pewaukee had to be sold. Julia was persuaded to move to Elmwood Place—a retirement community. She lived there for three years and adjusted to it well. She had her own apartment. She was mentally alert and would go out to wash her clothes or go for the one meal a day in the dining room. Julia got to know some ladies there and enjoyed their company. Julia liked that apartment mostly because she had her privacy. She could pass time on her own or with her family, when they were visiting. After her cognitive status declined to the extent that she could not take care of herself, she was relocated to the care home.

Brenda (as related by her daughter Betty)
Utica, New York

Brenda was born in Utica, New York, in 1906. Her father owned a shoe repair shop, where she worked as a child. The name of the shop was Brown's, and her grandfather had originally owned it. Brenda liked the smell of leather in the shop. There was a corner in the shop that had a wooden box where she used to keep her own work with leftover leather. There was a small window behind that corner that had a view of the alley. Brenda remembered the foggy window of that shop and how she used to draw things in the moisture of the window.

At the age of 21 she married Hank, and they moved to Worcester, Massachusetts. The houses in her neighborhood were called "triple-deckers": they had three floors, and each floor had separate apartments for three different families. The house in Worcester was special to Brenda. It had a picket fence and a huge yard with flowers everywhere. She liked to garden, as did her husband. They had flowers all along the fence. It was just lovely. They lived in that house for about nine years.

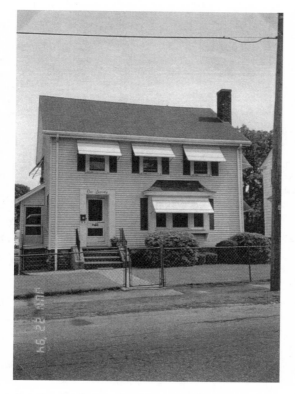

Brenda's first house after her marriage, in Worcester, Massachusetts. Brenda took the picture when she was visiting the house years after having moved away.

The Farm in Greenfield, Massachusetts

Brenda's husband had always talked about going into dairy farming, and finally they made the decision to buy a farm. They went to live on a farm in Greenfield, Massachusetts. She was unhappy about leaving her beautiful house in the city. That had been her own first house, where she had done a lot of things by herself, like putting new wallpaper in the kitchen, painting the bedrooms, and, especially, putting in the garden. But after a while she got used to farm life. She grew to love the place and the animals. She loved the cows and gave every cow a name. They all were

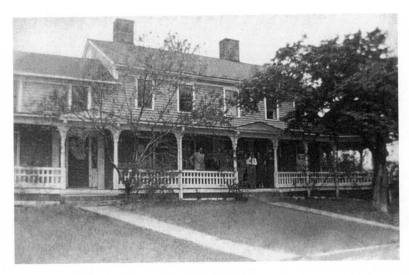

Brenda's family farm, in Greenfield, Massachusetts

individuals and special to her. She also raised vegetables for the family—tomatoes, cucumbers, and corn.

They had a huge tent, where all the equipment was kept. In the summers, the family would often sleep in the tent. Brenda liked staying in the tent. She thought that it was like a small world of her own with a sky that she could touch. They went camping often and slept in a tent. When the children became teenagers, the family stayed in cabins. They returned to the same place by the river every year. Hank went fishing every day, and Brenda rowed the boat while he fished. A river ran through their farm. Her husband fished in the river. There were mountains behind their home. The mountains were called either the Green Mountains or the White Mountains. There was also a big hay field behind the house. The deer often came down—herds of deer—to the edge of the cornfield or the hay field. Brenda was always fond of wildlife, so she watched closely to see when deer would be in the field. She wrote a poem about a deer and the cornfield.

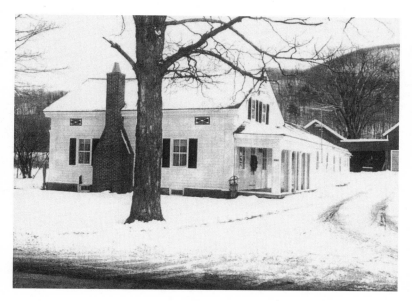

Brenda and Hank's farm, in New York

The Farm in New York

Five years later, Brenda and Hank bought another farm in upstate New York at the edge of the New York–Vermont state line. There were a lot of skiers in that area, and Brenda and Hank let some of them stay in one end of the house that wasn't used. The family slept upstairs over the main portion of the house. At one point Hank added on a wing with rooms that they then rented out to hunters on a regular basis.

Moving from the Farm

A few years later, Hank became very ill. He and Brenda couldn't take care of the farm any longer. So the farm was sold and the family moved back to Massachusetts. Hank died within a couple of years. At that point Brenda's daughter Amanda helped her mother move into an apartment not far from hers in Milwaukee. Brenda didn't like that apartment be-cause of the noise of traffic from the highway. After a year she moved to

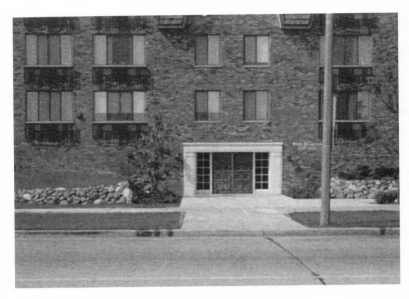

Brenda's final independent home, in Milwaukee, Wisconsin

another apartment down the street that was farther from the highway and closer to a park. Brenda went walking in the park every day. She said that the park reminded her of the open farms she had lived on before. She lived in that apartment for several years.

Gradually Brenda's health began to decline. Her daughter Amanda suggested that she move to an assisted living facility. Once Brenda was living there, her health stabilized. She worked as the building secretary for 10 years. At one point, her health worsened quickly and she wasn't able to take care of her apartment. Amanda came over to clean the place and took Brenda's laundry home and brought simple food that Brenda could still prepare. Eventually Brenda could no longer do anything, and she had started to forget things.

Home Stories and Guided Recollection

Can people with dementia remember their homes? Can prompts trigger recollection of past places? My experience in carrying out guided conversations with persons who have dementia gives positive answers to both questions. Individuals were able to remember and share more about their past when I used specific personal information as the basis for both verbal and visual prompts, especially photographs of home.

Using Prompts to Guide Reminiscence

As inducers of recollection, prompts, also referred to as *reminiscentia* (Sherman, 1995), can include photographs, letters, souvenirs, relics—any objects that are presumed to have some meaning to the older person. Personal photographs in particular are among the most cherished objects for residents in a care facility, and thus can be especially helpful for guided reminiscence.

A photograph is a wonderful thing. It allows us to pause, reflect, wonder, and remember. It helps us stand outside the flow of time because of its "stillness." Videos are too close to how we experience the world; therefore, they do not help us stop and think in the way photographs do. The personal photograph speaks a language of longing. It is not an object that arises out of material need or use value; it is an object arising out of the need to remember—or, rather, the psychological yearning for reminiscence. The subjective value of a photograph is embedded in the personal life experience attached to its origin and in the interpretation of the original experience that evolves over time. The photograph gains new dimensions of meaning with the life events of the person connected to it. In this, the meaning of a photograph is dynamic. Although a photograph represents a particular event and/or people captured in a moment, it has the potential to trigger a host of memories beyond the specific moment and event. Like a capsule that has compressed time, it can unlock memories of past experiences in vivid and real ways by the viewer. This is a fascinating dimension of the power of photos in going beyond the moments in time to a much larger set of events, people, and emotions. Moreover, the visual nature of photographs helps people to *visualize* the experience in a way that might be limited in other types of reminiscentia. As the visual aspect of experience is one of the most important sources of perception, it is natural that a visual aid can provide a bridge to the particular place and/or people in the photograph.

In guided conversations with nursing home residents with dementia, I used both generic place photographs and residents' personal photographs as prompts. Generic place types included the environments where the age cohort of the residents might have spent their childhood and adult years (i.e., homes, neighborhoods, urban streets, countryside, eating places, schoolhouses, work places, natural settings, etc., from the turn of the century to the 1960s). Personal photographs included those of the residents' past homes, places visited, and family events. In some cases I included photographs of personally meaningful artifacts (e.g., the car in which one resident had traveled or artwork created by the resident's mother that used to be displayed in her home).

The guided conversations took place in the resident's room in the care facility or in a common space (e.g., lounge, activity space, dining area). I would introduce myself and ask the resident how she was doing. I would then tell her that I wanted to talk about her life, especially about places in her life. To help the resident feel at ease, I talked briefly about the city where I grew up, the homes I remember, and how these memories sometimes come back to me, and asked casual questions of the resident indicating a reciprocal interest in knowing her life story. So as I talked about my childhood home, I asked, "Do you remember the home you grew up in?" Sharing parts of my own "home story" helped residents relate to the kind of response I was looking for.

When I simply asked questions (e.g., Do you remember the home from your childhood? Do you remember anything about the neighborhood where you lived as a child?), residents' responses were disjointed and did not go beyond their birth year and place. However, once I began to use verbal and visual prompts to share specific information about their past, residents were able to recollect and share more. For example, I would say, "You know what, Helen? I know your daughter, and I talked with her today about you. She told me that you grew up in Chippewa Falls and that you were living on a farm. Do you remember that place?" As these personal prompts helped them to connect and retrieve from memory, mentioning the resident's daughter or son also enabled her relate to me as a "friend," someone who could be trusted. In these first conversations I focused on using verbal prompts of information gathered from family members; in later conversations I focused on using photographs and artwork as prompts. Not surprisingly, most of the residents I spoke with were unable to retrieve memories of places from their adult years. When asked about homes or other significant places from that stage in their lives, residents usually either related something pertaining to their childhood home or did not communicate coherently. But most could recollect —sometimes vividly—memories linked to places in their early lives, their childhood schools, and, for some, the homes of their early adult years.

Early Places

The topic of early places primarily involved remembering about early childhood places as opposed to places known in adulthood. For example, Julia remembered the address of the house where she grew up. As she recalled the address, she also remembered positively her family and friends:

Julia: Nine fifteen 17th Street

Q: And which town was that?

Julia: . . . that's New London, Wisconsin. It was a nice place . . . It wasn't large at that time. But everybody helped each other. That's all I can tell you.

When I prompted Julia about her childhood days at her grandparents' farm in Nebraska, she seemed to react quickly to the cue and recalled the activity of walking to get the mail. Her immediate recollection of getting the mail points that out as a pleasant activity for her. Once again, her appreciation of the contacts with neighbors/friends is consistent with her positive memories of family at her home in New London.

Q: How about Springfield, Nebraska?

Julia: Yes, we were there. My grandparents were farmers there, and we'd go there in the summertime. I used to love to walk back and forth to get the mail. We had to walk about a half a mile to get it. But it was fun to do because I'd see people and they'd say, "Hi, Julie," and things like that. That was nice.

Joyce was more "reserved" than Julia and had more difficulty recalling earlier places. I had interviewed her son Stephen to gather information about her. She could remember the date of her birth but needed a prompt for the place:

Q: I talked with your son, Stephen, and he told me a little bit about your life. I would also like to hear from you. Do you remember when you were born?

Joyce: On the nineteenth of November.

Q: Which year was that?

Joyce: I don't, just right off now, I don't remember.

Q: How about the place of your birth?

Joyce: Somewhere north, I think.

Q: You were born in Vernon County, Wisconsin?

Joyce: Yeah, uh-huh. Vernon County, sure. How can I forget?

Q: Do you remember anything about the house itself, where you were living?

Joyce: Yeah.

Q: What was it like?

Joyce: It was a brick house. And we had a nice house. There was a porch, and one day my father brought a swing chair. I liked it very much. And then we had the farm that we got along on. I worked on the farm—taking care of the animals, keeping the place clean. So that, where we lived, it was on the ridge. Everybody went for that, you know, wanted to stay there, where they didn't want to leave. We were not rich, but the life was good.

As I showed Joyce a generic picture, she recalled the farm and her grandparents' home on that farm. She used the house in the picture as a reference point to describe physical locations (e.g., her family house, grandparents' house, lawn, barn and shed on the remembered farm):

My grandpa and grandma lived in a house like that. Our house was kind of close there to the road. And then we built another, smaller house for Grandpa and Grandma. Then we had to take care of the milk. We had that. Another lawn, and then we had a big barn. And after that, we got a shed, built a shed, and chicken coop, and pig barn. It was all. So we got along.

Maria could remember the date and place of her birth by herself:

Q: Do you remember when you were born? What year was that?

Maria: Nineteen fourteen.

Q: What month was that?

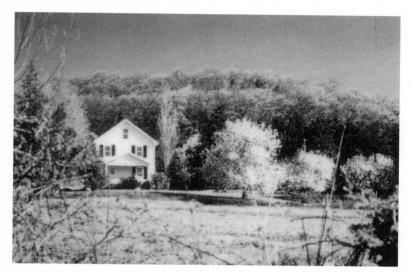

Generic picture of a farm

Maria: June, June 14th, I was born, 1914.
Q: And where was that? Where were you born?
Maria: Menomonie, Wisconsin.

Based on my interview with her daughter Rebecca, I prompted Maria with the Web house, an important family home. She remembered that the house had been built by her grandfather and that she and her cousin had gone there often. As she described the place, she expressed a desire to go back and visit:

Q: Do you remember about the Web house?
Maria: That's in Menomonie. My grandpa built that. My aunt is still living in there. So we used to go down there, like on Sundays, and spend time with her or her relatives. So my cousin Liz and I, we used to go down there. Yes, he built it. It had an old barn in the back. And he planted trees and all kinds of things. I think my aunt is still there. I would like to visit her again. I think the place is still there.
Q: Did you go to the Web house often?
Maria: Almost every Sunday. My aunt's daughter is from Eau Claire, is crippled, and so they took the car and go from Eau Claire down to

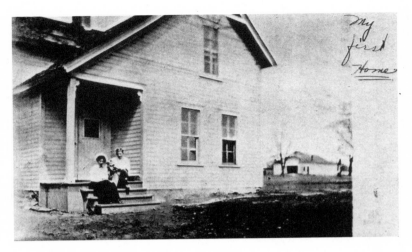

Maria's family home, in Menomonie, Wisconsin

Menomonie to visit them because Margaret couldn't walk very good, and she wanted to go out.

Personal photographs were also helpful in aiding Maria's recollection of places from her past. Although she was somewhat noncommunicative in the beginning, as she looked at the photographs she began to talk as if it were all coming back to her. The quiet Maria became verbal as she described her childhood home, as though she were seeing the place in her mind. Her speech was coherent, and her eyes were focused as she recognized and recalled her first family home in Menomonie:

Maria: Yes, that's us in Menomonie. And this is my dad and my mother. He was a caretaker of the fairgrounds. He took care of the grounds and all that stuff. I was only four years old at that time. My mother used to sit on the steps every day. My dad was very loving. He used to walk from the fairgrounds office about two miles away from our home. My mother used to sit on the steps and wait for my dad in the afternoon. You could see the road for quite a distance from our steps. I used to pass the fairgrounds on my way to school.

Q: You probably went to the fairs, too?

Maria: Sure. It was the Northern Wisconsin State Fair, and there wasn't

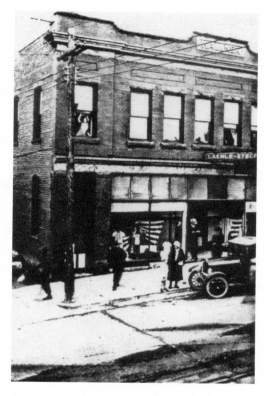

Uncle Joe's apartment, in Eau Claire, Wisconsin,
where Maria and her brother stayed for some time

any fairs around. So lot of people were coming there. Eau Claire is
close by, and that was a bigger town than Menomonie. It was a big
event in Menomonie.

Maria also recognized a photograph of her aunt and uncle's apartment
building:

*That's in Park Falls. My brother and I lived with my aunt for some time.
That was a busy street, Division Street. I used to like the parades on the
street. There were big windows from upstairs, and I could see the people and
cars from the room where I slept. There was a grocery store downstairs
owned by my aunt and uncle. My aunt across the street was very good to us.*

She raised my father because his mother died when he was four. And she was very good to us.

Homes are located in neighborhoods, and neighborhoods are in towns or cities. Depending on the specific urban context, a city can make a lasting impression on one's memory. Although the environmental scale of a city is different from that of a home, the emotional attachment can be equally strong. For example, Mary was more interested in sharing her memories of the city than memories of any of her homes. New York City had a distinct appeal in her recollection of the past:

Q: What do you remember about your childhood home?

Mary: Everything. I was born in Manhattan. My whole life was in Manhattan until I got married. Oh, you know, Manhattan Island, that's New York. It's an island, so you got a lot of water around there. The river's there and all. It's a beautiful site. My sister lives on the 28th floor in Manhattan. So when you go up to her house, to her apartment, you go into the dining room and you see one side of Manhattan. Then you go through all the apartment, you see all of this. It's really beautiful. Well, like here, when you go to a high-rise and you see the whole section, the rooms, you're impressed. It's either higher or lower, or whatever. The thing that people like most is the city and Empire State Building. Then when they had that crash, on the Empire State Building, whoever came to New York, that's the first thing they wanted to see. But you could see there was something there. But it didn't take long. They had it all built up already. And the Woolworth Building was the highest building at the time. I just love that city.

Although Mary had not mentioned much about her home in New York City, when prompted with generic pictures she later remembered some physical characteristics of the kitchen in her childhood home. For example, a picture of a kitchen reminded her of the kitchen in her early home. Even as she described the kitchen, her recollections took her back to her liking for the city:

That's like our kitchen. We had the refrigerator there. And, of course, the stove. And we had—let's see, our kitchen wasn't as elaborate as this here.

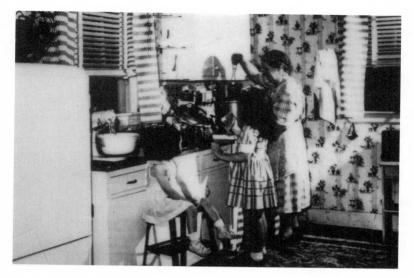

Generic picture of a kitchen

But there they use it, like my mother's house. It wasn't pretentious, but opposite the kitchen is like a breakfast room. There really is, you eat there, your meals there. Then the dining room. You utilize that. But then they had kitchens there from years ago that was beautiful. You know, I can't describe things to you. They had the refrigerator and then like between here and there a wall, and so then in between would be a little table, just for little snacks. We had a good view of the neighborhood street from our kitchen window. Well, it was, I'll tell you, it was a close, a close-knit neighborhood. The Jewish people lived together, and the Christians lived separately. It was a nice area. Well, neighborhoods are much more alive in New York City.

Meredith was silent when I started talking without giving any prompts. She was withdrawn and apparently not interested in talking. However, when I shared some photographs that I had collected from her daughter, Meredith's outlook changed dramatically. She was visibly moved by the photographs and was teary-eyed as she remembered her childhood:

Oh, that's interesting! That's my old home where I was born and raised— Ahmeek Street. Oh, that's interesting. That's surprising. You sat across the street and took those. Ahmeek Street. That was what they call a double

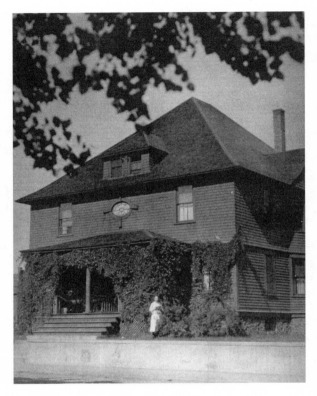

Meredith standing in front of her childhood home in Michigan

house, two houses together. That's in upper Michigan, and these are the vines on our front porch. We called them—and they were so beautiful, so pretty. Yes, it was lovely, just loved it. The porch was just beautiful. You could look out the window and see these beautiful vines on the front porch, looking through the inside window outside. There were, like, four or five stairwells, and each of the stairwells had a storage room under the stairs, and when you were inside one of those and shut the door, it was very dark. You couldn't tell which house or which stairwell you were in. It was very comfortable. I liked it very, very much. Six rooms on each side. And the—six rooms upstairs and down, or six rooms in the whole house, I guess. It was a home I enjoyed, enjoyed having company visit me, too.

Meredith also recalled her cousin, with whom she was apparently close. For her, memories of the double house were intertwined with memories of her mother and her mother's twin sister:

> They used to call them double houses up there, at that time, and they were, my mother and her twin sister, so the twin sisters lived in the same house. And they're always close friends. And her daughter and me were very close. So we were close. We went to parochial school, high school and grade school. Grade school and high school. They called me and my cousin sisters, twins—like my mother and her sister—and like the double house. I guess we are all meant to be in that double house.

Memories of School

As residents recollected their early years, memories of school life came through as a natural consequence. For some, recollections of schooldays emerged without specific questions. For others, they were triggered by suggestive questions or verbal/visual prompts. For example, Teresa could recollect bits and pieces of her school as I prompted her with the name of her childhood hometown:

Q: Do you remember anything about Grafton?

Teresa: I remember about that quite often. When I think of it, I think of things I've done there, where I've gone to school.

Q: What do you remember about the school?

Teresa: Well, first I went to Lutheran school. Then I went to—I don't remember. We had to walk about a half a mile to our school. We had an eighth-grade education. Well, it was just an ordinary school. We had all the different classes in there, from first to fourth grade. And we had geography and history, and reading and writing. "Reading and writing and 'rithmetic, taught to the tune of a hickory stick." If you knew that song. They never sent me to high school or anything like that. But I remember the river close to that school. I'll never forget that because once we went out and took pictures. Oh boy, that was a big deal at that time.

Janet could also recall the walk to her school in Milwaukee. For Janet, school was more interesting because of the walk to and from home. The activities on the street and talking with friends were good reasons to go to school:

Q: Janet, did you go to West Division High School?

Janet: Sure, I did. How do you know that? I used to walk to that school, seven blocks from our home. It was west of us, about seven blocks or something like that. I don't know exactly. It was West Division High School, that's what it was. West Division. West Division High School. That's where I went. I don't know if they all went to it. But that's where I went to high school. When we were real little, we probably went with my sister, but afterwards, we went ourselves. My friend Nancy and I walked together. We would pass the State Bank blue building, a bridge over the river, and the alley. That was always dark, and we saw mice running one day. I guess. But I liked the walk to school. I think I had my own time with my friend talking about all kinds of things and enjoying the neighborhood.

One the other hand, Meredith did not say anything about her school until she saw a picture of it. This was the one-room schoolhouse where she studied in Michigan, where her aunt was the teacher:

Q: Does this look familiar?

Meredith: It looks like the school I went to. Oh my, it is that school. Is it real? I think I can remember now. It was just one great big room. There were over 20 children in there, over 20. I don't know just how many. But there were more than 20 children that went to school there. "You wrote on your slate, 'I love you, Joe,' when we were a couple of kids." The boys and girls were in the same room. But they sat on one side, and the girls sat on the other side. We had, I would say, up to the fourth grade. They had a playground on the school, where we could play during the recess. We could play hide and seek. We would hide behind the schoolhouse or hide in the toilet or something. Then the folks didn't send me to high school.

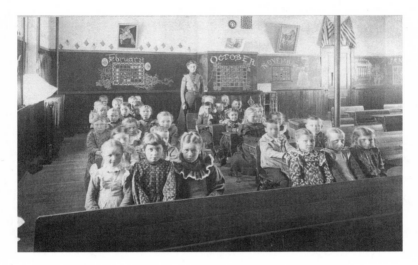

Inside the one-room schoolhouse in Michigan where Meredith studied

Homes in Early Adult Years

In general, the residents I conversed with seemed able to recall childhood homes and other places with less effort than their homes of later years. Fewer residents offered recollections of places from their adult years, and all were triggered by verbal and visual prompts.

For instance, responding to verbal prompts, Sheila could remember the cottage she and her husband had. At times during our conversation she would say that the cottage was still there and that she visited the place often (Sheila did not have any family member in town, and apart from the facility's occasional in-town field trips, she had not left the nursing home for the past two years). At other times she would say matter-of-factly that the cottage was gone. Her emotional attachment to the cottage was reflected in her desire to visit the place and in an expression of loss:

> Q: You had a cottage by the River Escanaba. Can you tell me about that cottage?
>
> Sheila: Oh, yes. I had a cottage, I still have that cottage on the river. I visited the place just the other day.
>
> Q: What is it like? Describe the cottage.

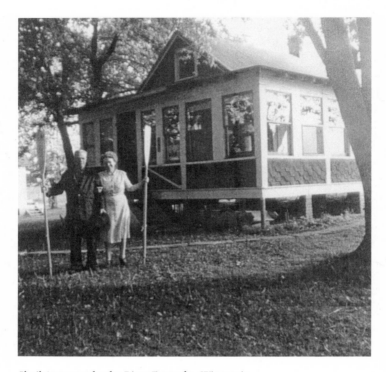

Sheila's cottage by the River Escanaba, Wisconsin

Sheila: The cottage? It was just an ordinary one, great big living room
and two bedrooms. That's about it. And a kitchen. It had a kitchen
and a big porch halfway around both sides like that.

Q: That sounds nice.

Sheila: Yeah. Oh, the cottage was very nice. I still own it. I'll be going
there next weekend.

Q: Here's a picture of the cottage.

Sheila: Oh, that is our cottage! Yeah, it had fish-scale wooden sidings.
The cottage was made of wood. We had a large wood on the farm,
and Father had a lot of lumber cut. I used to call it "the fish house."
Oh, we went fishing on the river. Oh, we got the biggest fish. I don't
remember getting a larger fish. Oh, we did get one large fish. What
the heck was it called, now? Bullhead. We went fishing at night, and
we caught bullheads. Do you know what bullheads are?

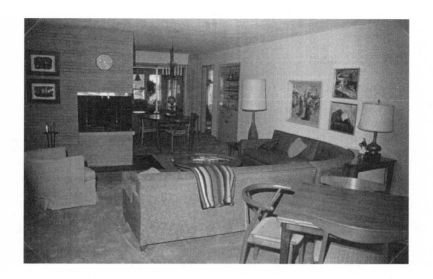

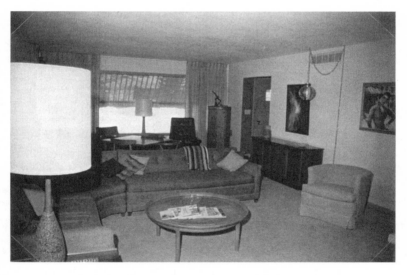

Interior images of Julia's home (pictures taken by Julia's husband)

Q: No.

Sheila: They don't have scales. They have skin, you got to skin 'em. They were good to eat.

Q: You like going to the cottage?

Sheila: Oh, yes. I used to go there and stay there all summer and then come back to my house, to my father and mother, in the winter. I don't know whether my first cottage is there anymore or not. I'd have to ask my family, I guess, my nephew, it is disappeared or not. But it seems to me it disappeared with the water, the river. I liked that cottage very much. I think I have lost a valuable [piece].

For Julia, the feeling of losing a home was expressed as "closing" the place. According to her daughter, Julia was a "homebody," and she took much pride in her home. I showed her photographs of the house taken by her husband, who loved the house as well. She recognized those pictures as being of her home:

Q: Julia, take a look at this picture.

Julia: My house in Pewaukee. Yes, that's where we lived for a long time. And then they closed it. There wasn't any more.

Q: So, they closed it.

Julia: They didn't have to. I was living there, and I took care of it. We got those lamps from a store in our neighborhood. Oh, that sofa was from my in-laws. My husband didn't want to take it out. And I said to him, "You have things, and so do I." There was a picture frame of a farm that I got from my grandma. I think she did it herself. All of this is gone. The place was closed.

For Teresa, letting go of her cottage on Pickerel Lake was like letting go of a close friend. She talked about the cottage as a "somebody" who comforted her not only when she was staying there during the summer but also at other times. Like Julia and Sheila, she couldn't recall anything about this place from her early adulthood when prompted by only generic questions, but she was able to remember after looking at the photograph:

Q: Teresa, your daughter was telling me about a cottage you had. Do you remember anything about that?

Teresa: Maybe. I don't know.

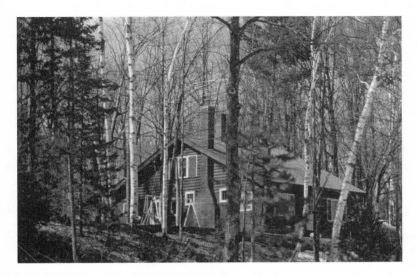

Teresa's cottage, on Pickerel Lake, upper Michigan

Q: This picture may help you remember.

Teresa: Oh, yes. I hated to give it up.

Q: Why? You liked it?

Teresa: I don't know, just giving it up.

Q: Uh-huh.

Teresa: It was something I hated to do. I hated to give it up because it was a friend.

Q: It was a friend?

Teresa: Yeah, it happened over the years. It was a beautiful cottage. Beautiful lake. We had a good time there for part of summers.

Q.: What kinds of things did you do while you were there?

Teresa: Well, regular things, you know. I felt each time I was there—it was like meeting your good friend. It gave me comfort. I felt good. I didn't like Milwaukee. But it felt good that I will be going to the cottage in May.

All these memories are emotionally colored. Julia describes how she "used to love to walk back and forth" to get the mail on her grandparents' farm. A family photograph reminds Maria of how loving her father was.

Mary remembers the "beautiful" kitchen she had in Manhattan and describes the neighborhoods there as "more alive." Teresa recalls her summer cottage as "like meeting your good friend." What emerges from these memories is the emotional tone of the remembered activity or place.

Holding On to Feelings

Emotions form an important part of our lives and, consequently, of our memories. These conversations reveal how autobiographical memories are shaped by the emotional intensity and personal significance of an event or place. From this perspective, there are no life experiences devoid of emotion. Although we don't yet fully understand the complex, multifaceted relationship between cognition and emotion, there is some evidence that emotions are precursors of cognitive processes; in other words, there cannot be a cognitive experience without the triggering of an emotional experience as well. Alternatively, some have suggested that cognition and emotion are interrelated, an intertwined system that under certain circumstances can allow emotional processes to function independently. In either view, the depth of emotion varies across various life experiences, making some events more "neutral" and others more "emotional."

As we recall positive or negative life experiences, the associated emotions are regenerated. So a person recalling pleasant times from his or her childhood is likely to feel good. As we recreate our experiences in the process of reminiscing, the affective dimensions of the original experience are reconstructed in keeping with the individual's strength of recall, personal characteristics, and present psychosocial condition. Positive memories seem to be more accessible than neutral memories, more detailed, and comparatively resistant to forgetting.

In our conversations, residents with dementia expressed loss and yearning for past homes. But the process of recollecting places from the past was an activity most of the residents were willing to participate in. Many commented that they felt good talking about past places and events. From this standpoint, the process of reminiscing seemed to have a positive effect, even though the actual recollection may have been emotional. For instance, Julia was visibly distressed when she recalled the experience of moving out of her house before coming to the nursing home. She had

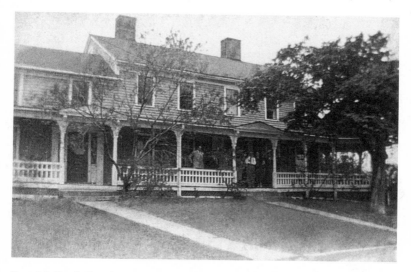

Brenda's family farmhouse, in Greenfield, Massachusetts

mentioned earlier how much pride she took in the house and how much she enjoyed doing things in it. Here she expresses her sense of loss as a present-day reality that she is holding on to:

Q: What was it like to move out of that home?

Julia: I hated to move out of it. Nice place. That's the last house I was in. Nice place.

Q: Why did you hate it? Because you liked it so much?

Julia: Well, they had to close it because they didn't have any more money to have it. The home was my life, and I left behind everything in that home. I have to live with that now. What can I do?

Brenda reacted similarly when she saw the photograph of her family farmhouse. Her emotional attachment to the farm was reflected in her words in a positive way, with no hint of loss. In a controlled and measured way, she shared some of her feelings:

Q: Brenda, does this picture remind you of anything?

Brenda: Our farm in Greenfield, Massachusetts. I lost that picture. That's an apple tree, and that's the long porch.

Q: It does seem to be a long porch.

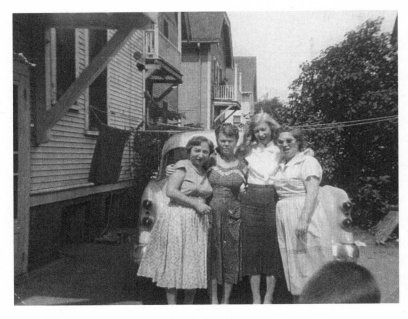

Pauline, her sister, and friends in her backyard

Brenda: Yeah, we'd sit there on the front and we'd talk, in the summertime. In the winter, of course, we didn't do that. But we kept that
picture because I liked it. I wanted to enlarge it. Was that last year?
Maybe the year before. I lost the picture. The farm life was good. It
was hard work, but good life.

Q: What else comes to your mind about the farm?

Brenda: It's right in front of me—I can see my father and my brother
Jim working on the field. I used to work around the house with my
sister Jane. It was a good life. My life was very good on the farm.

For Pauline, memories of place were closely intertwined with memories of her family. Talking about her family home, she was expressive
about her love for her grandmother and her sister. Her feelings about
her family members were embedded in her memories of her childhood
home. Looking at a photograph of herself, her sister, and some friends,
she recalled:

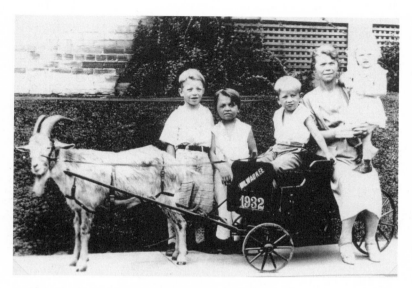

Pauline with friends in her childhood neighborhood

Pauline: Well, I'll tell you, I'm trying to remember. It's a few years now. Well, it was—we didn't have the luxuries, but it was a good house. And my grandma did the cooking. See, my mother died, so my grandmother raised my sister and me. So we got along very well. The house here was my grandma's. Grandma took good care of the place and we helped her . . . I love my grandma very much and my sister. We were three people in that house. I had a good time in grandma's place. Sometimes I want to go back. See, when you have love from the family, then you don't miss your home very much.

Q: Do you recognize anybody in this picture [a photograph of some children with a goat-cart]?

Pauline: . . . These are cousins. This is my little brother. This is my little sister. Oh, for God—1932. Oh, my God in heaven. That's my little brother. Oh, God in heaven. Where did you get these? I love them so much. That's in Grandma's neighborhood back street. We always played there. I love them so much.

As Linda talked about her childhood home, her emotions were clear. Her eyes became teary and her voice muffled. Linda was clearly remem-

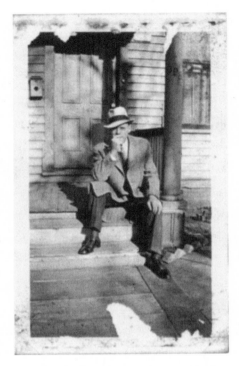

Linda's father sitting on the front porch of
her childhood home

bering the past as past and expressed her wish to visit her home again. She
was moved to see the photographs that I had borrowed from her niece,
visibly excited and emotionally moved. At one point she stopped talking,
sat in her wheelchair, and quietly wept. Then she spoke:

> *That's my dad sitting on the steps of our home on the south side.* I miss my
> home so much. *When my brother was living, before he was married and
> stuff, he'd come and stay with us. That's our home, that's our only home. I
> love my dad. He used to play with me and my brother in the yard. There was
> no grass and there was a swing. That's it. I can't help it. I guess it's natural. I
> don't know* . . . And, I want to go back and see our home once more
> before I leave the earth. I just want to go down once more and visit my
> home. That's all.

In these conversations, verbal and visual prompts were effective tools for reminiscence in several ways. First, in most cases they successfully jogged residents' memories and elicited at least some recollection compared with general conversation about the past. Although most of the residents I spoke with could not articulate their past in a coherent way in response to generic questions, the same individuals were able to recall and share more after looking at personal photographs or in response to my verbal prompts with information regarding their past places. Second, even when the recollections triggered were substantively "sketchy" or disjointed, the prompts were invaluable in their capacity to arouse a "recollective" state of mind in which the individual may or may not share the place experience in a narrative form but nevertheless relives the experience in its emotional connotations. Finally, the personal items were instrumental in creating rapport between the residents and me. As they came to know that I knew their family members (in most cases, a daughter or son) and had the photographs with me, I came to be considered a "friend." This rapport helped them to be at ease with me, feel less threatened in conversation, and open up to the possibility of sharing personal experiences.

Personal Prompts as Triggers for Recollection

The selection of pictures or verbal prompts based on information gathered from family members is subject to both functional limitations and second-generation interpretation. For example, if no photograph is available of a particular home to which a resident was emotionally attached, there may be a missed opportunity for triggering her recollection about that particular home. Also, the decision about which photographs family members share are colored by their interpretations, which may or may not coincide with residents' subjective past experiences. Thus, conversations with residents who have dementia can be limited to or shaped by the family members' added layers of interpretation.

The presence of such "contextual" aspects suggests that residents' memories of places involve a complex and layered process of recreation. The process I observed among the residents and family members I spoke with is typical: originally a particular resident with dementia shared memories with her family member. Those memories were carried and further shaped by the family member's own interpretation of the events as well as his or her personal attitudes, belief, and preferences. In recounting their loved one's place stories, family members may have added another layer of interpretation or meaning. Finally, as I used fragments of these stories as prompts, the resident revisited the memories within the current reality of his or her disease. That is, the recollecting of places is a dynamic and evolving reality. Thus, for these residents with dementia, recollection reflects a process of "re-collecting" past place experiences via several of the above-mentioned steps. The process of guided reminiscence was a creative one in which family members, the residents, and I collected fragments of the individuals' memories and put them together. By themselves, residents' responses don't reveal the complex, multidimensional process that links recollections with family memories and family members' subjective recounting.

Emergent Present

In guided conversations that elicit residents' memories of home as ways to reach beyond the disease to the person, it is not only the past that can be meaningful. For a person with dementia, the temporal boundaries of past, present, and future are blurred. Our taken-for-granted linear temporal categories become indistinct; the mind regresses to childhood, and the future becomes the moment at hand. Perhaps in this temporal shift the significance of the present gains an added dimension. It is "now," the present, that endears the past and creates the future, and in this process the present becomes eternal. From this perspective, present time is emergent in the context of the personal reality of "living in the past" as well as the sociopsychological reality of life in a nursing home.

As I tried to elicit residents' impressions about their personal present in nursing homes and what the future might hold for them, the general response was one of acceptance and taking one day at a time. Some residents talked about the positive aspects of life in terms of specific issues, while others seemed to create a more abstract and philosophical grounding for their lives in the nursing homes. For instance, Janet was pragmatic in her characterization of her life and mentioned the "goodness" of her facility. She seemed reasonably content with the routine of her life. When I asked her how she felt about the current place, her response was:

> Well, I, it depends upon how my feeling is. If I have a pretty good place to stay, and you can't find something every day . . . So you can't go looking at a hundred different places. You take what comes along, that's all. So, I do have some friends here now. The food is good. They take care of me. This is good life for me.

Linda was among the more cognitively aware residents and was able to articulate her recollections of the past as well as her thoughts about life in the nursing home. With a rather philosophical attitude, she recognized that there was no choice for her, accepted her situation as something of a *fait accompli*. And in this acceptance of the situation as being part of her destiny, she was probably better able to cope. In Linda's words:

> I have no choice. No longer would they let me live in there. But I just would like to look at the whole home, the way it is, and the yard now, you know. But otherwise, everything is good here. There's nothing wrong with being here. It's fine as a home, and it is a home, and a very good one. But not like your own. You get what I mean? You know, you gotta be somewhere. So here I am. Not much, cause I'm really toward the end—you know, 90. Ninety is 90. I don't know how much longer I'll be around. I don't keep track of time. I am okay.

Lisa could remember only bits and pieces about her home after marriage. She smiled when she said a few times, "I don't remember well." She seemed to be alert to her present circumstances and could describe some of the activities that took place on the unit. Although she was clearly not able to remember anything coherent from her past, she was happy with the present. For her, life was in the real present, and her life in the nursing home was what mattered. The past and future seemed irrelevant. Lisa was articulate in present time:

> I don't remember well. That was long time back. I am doing fine here. They have some activities I go to. The rabbi comes once every week; I like his talk. I have friends here. This is just fine. You are always fine.

Using Home Stories to Build Caregiving Relationships

Home stories can help persons with dementia sustain—even recapture, in some measure—a sense of self. Using photographs of home, along with life narratives emerging from individuals' own memories and family members' or friends' recollections of stories and memories their loved ones have shared, can benefit persons with dementia in two ways. First, such guided reminiscence can anchor residents in remembered places, activities, and events even as their disease threatens to leave them adrift in a present they may no longer fully understand. Even when particular recollections prompt strong emotional responses, the process of reminiscing can have positive effects. Second, home stories can enable caregivers to better understand and engage residents *as persons*. By making visible to the staff the homes residents have known, the textures of the lives they have lived in specific and remembered places, home stories can provide opportunities for caregivers to have more effective interactions with residents. That will enhance not only residents' quality of life but also caregivers' professional satisfaction and morale.

CHAPTER FIVE

Home Work

Putting Home Stories to Work in Dementia Care

> Care is concerned primarily with the maintenance and
> enhancement of personhood. Providing a safe environment,
> meeting basic needs and giving physical care are all essential,
> but only part of the care of the whole person.
>
> —*Tom Kitwood*, Dementia Reconsidered *(1997)*

There is growing recognition that it is critical to *recognize, validate, and work with* the whole person in dementia care (Kitwood, 1997; Sabat, 2002, 2001; Hughes et al., 2006). The task-oriented culture of traditional dementia care must transform into a person-centered culture in which the conditions and behavioral challenges of dementia are not ignored but rather are addressed with a comprehensive understanding of the person and his or her uniqueness, past life experience, and present situation. Because verbal communication is challenging, it is important to connect through gestures and expressions that relate to the person's emotional sensibilities. Although the reality of the front-line workers in dementia care is shaped by the immediate demands of numerous tasks—feeding the person, dressing the person, getting the charts done—it is imperative that we step back and revisit the personal and organizational values and priorities that affect the quality of interaction with the person who has dementia.

Psychologist Tom Kitwood argued the importance of the "person" with dementia and pioneered recognition of the concept of personhood as central to dementia care, noting that personhood "is a standing or status that is bestowed on one human being, by others, in the context of relation-ship and social being. It implies recognition, respect and trust" (Kitwood, 1997, p. 8). Personhood is in part a social relational concept, meaning that the ways in which others interact with or respond to a person who has dementia support that person's sense of self. The ways in which the per-son is treated with dignity, love, and caring and is valued as a human being contribute to the social context of personhood. At a more funda-mental level, as indicated in chapters 1 and 2, the understanding of a person should be grounded in the transcendent self that is beyond memo-ries, cognition, and emotions. Achieving a person-centered culture of dementia care requires that we strive to connect with the person who is *there,* no matter what the outer reality of disability might be. This is the ethical foundation of relating to the person as a human being.

Memories of homes and other meaningful places from a person's past can be valuable resources in caring for that individual. Home stories and personal *reminiscentia* help give recognition to the personhood of some-one who has dementia. By enabling caregivers to engage the individual's remaining memories, cognitive abilities, and—more important—emo-tions, home stories provide a key medium for relating to the individual's reality. Memories of the physical home become the means to connect to and help meet the individual's need to be *at home,* to be psychologically secure and comforted. This crucial connection can be achieved through conversations using personal verbal and visual prompts. Home is impor-tant not so much because it is more likely to be remembered than other places or experiences, but because memories of the place the individual has lived are more likely to reveal what home means for that person, whether as a physical place, an experience, or people in her or his life.

Although there is no empirical study examining the possible negative effect of remembering home for some persons with dementia, the staff members need to be alert to the possibility. For some residents, remem-bering home may be too emotional and could lead to "negative" behav-iors. In this study, a few residents occasionally became emotional and expressed a desire to "go home." However, their desire to go home did not lead to any other activity, such as wandering or trying to leave the unit. If such a situation does arise with any person, the conversation should be ended with a positive distraction. It is possible that home-related remembering may not be suitable for some individuals, who may become upset whenever any such conversation is initiated. As with any other reminiscence activity involving persons with dementia, sessions on home need to be conducted carefully, with an eye to the possibility of provoking distress. This cautionary note not withstanding, home stories have the potential to be useful resources for helping staff connect with the person who has dementia.

Using Home Stories to Enhance Care and Quality of Life

One of my objectives in interviewing family members of residents with dementia was to explore the value of residents' home stories for use by staff members on dementia care units. To explore this question, I developed home stories for several residents, including photographs, and surveyed nursing and activity staff members' perceptions and thoughts about how the home stories might help increase their knowledge about the residents and in turn be a resource for activities and social interaction. I shared these home stories with caregivers and through focus groups and an open-ended questionnaire invited them to reflect on how the stories might be useful in planning activities, what format the stories might take, where it might be useful to post stories in the facility, and so on. Their responses suggested four ways in which home stories might enhance care for persons with dementia: as tools for planning and carrying out activities, as aids for understanding behavior, as prompts for conversation, and as a means of promoting greater empathy in interactions with residents. Focus group sessions in particular helped identify practical guidance for developing and using home stories in dementia care.

Home Stories as Activity Tools

The life stories of residents with dementia in care facilities have shown promise for care planning and practice (Moos & Bjorn, 2006). Activities sensitively designed to match and capitalize on individual residents' former interests, preferences, and activities may be more meaningful than generic activities designed for any and all residents. Home stories thus should offer a powerful resource for the staff in developing targeted activities that residents may better relate to. Survey responses indicated that staff members felt home stories would be valuable in individual reminiscence sessions and small-group activities. An activities director noted:

> *Very valuable for activity staff to know background information such as this, because it helps us in programming especially in 1:1 situation. Helps staff to direct question to resident when reminiscing with resident.*

Activities can be more meaningful for persons with dementia when caregivers and family members are involved in a joint effort. In fact, collecting biographical knowledge and putting the information to work may provide an avenue for collaborative projects between staff and family. As one staff member pointed out:

> *This is a great way to involve families. Many family members want to be more involved, and we don't always have things to do together. Working on a resident's place-biosketch [home story] can be an interesting way to involve the families. In fact, this way we can know the families better.*

Staff members commented that generic activities can engage a few residents, but there are some residents who rarely participate in any activity. However, staff experience indicates that an activity the person had done in her or his past has much more appeal and is more likely to elicit interest. A few home stories included descriptions of the residents' daily activities in and around the home. Knowledge of those activities or lifestyle habits would be a useful tool for the staff. One response in this regard was:

> *We need to know the lifestyle activities of our residents. What did Mrs. _____ use to do in her homes all her life? She was a homemaker, so I am sure she spent a lot of time in the home. If I could know that, I could create an opportunity for her in the unit.*

Understanding Behaviors

Staff members believed that one of the potential benefits of knowing a resident's personal past is that it helps them understand the person's present actions/behaviors. For example, at Sunrise Nursing Home the staff always had a difficult time giving showers to a resident named Betty. She wouldn't cooperate in having the shower and often would become "irritated" and "depressed." Her home story, based on an interview with a niece who lives outside the state, revealed that Betty's sister Ann was a Holocaust survivor. Betty and Ann were close before Ann passed away, and Ann's experience in the concentration camps had apparently become part of Betty's memory. Although Betty herself had not experienced those terrible times, the word *shower* generated a manifest fear in her. One the nurses on the unit where Betty lived pointed out:

> *It helps the staff to know the background of the residents so they can understand some of the actions of residents and know how to better deal with their problems.*

As children, we typically engage in various play activities in and around the home and the neighborhood. It is not uncommon for some residents to experience themselves as in childhood, and they may try to relate to the environment in a manner typical of when they were children. Knowing about the person's childhood through her home, neighborhood, or school can help the staff gain an understanding of behavior that might otherwise appear strange or problematic, as we can see from this remark by a care aide:

> *This resident can all of a sudden decide to go under her bed. She was not upset, but we did not know how to react to her behavior . . . When I read her story, it said that she used to love going into this tiny space under the stairs in her home when she was seven to eight years old. I guess this was something she had mentioned to her daughter who is not in town. I think now I know why she may be going under the bed occasionally . . . This is harmless fun for her!*

Home Stories as Prompts for Conversation

Familiarity with residents' home stories provides a common ground for conversation between the staff and residents. Staff members often get to know about residents' families, hometowns, and significant people through informal conversations with those residents who can communicate and with their families. However, a resident with dementia may not be able to articulate her past well, and sometimes key family members live in distant cities or states, making it difficult if not impossible to collect residents' life histories. Several staff members mentioned that home stories could provide information that they could use to strike up conversations with residents who have dementia. Understanding a person's stories is the first step in developing a friendship. As a social worker responded:

You get to know the residents, and maybe you will have something in common with them to talk about. You can bring things up, and she can tell you how things were and tell you how they did them. It helps them enjoy talking about their lives that were so important to them.

Creating and Supporting Empathy

Individuals who have dementia can sometimes be noisy, hostile, aggressive, disruptive, violent, and nonconforming. Some are withdrawn and silent. Providing care for such people is at times highly demanding, and empathy can be hard to muster, especially in long-term care environments. Staff members' responses to home stories suggest, however, that such stories may be an important way to help create and sustain empathy for residents with dementia.

Empathy relates to having some understanding of what another person may be experiencing, gaining a glimpse of what life might be like from the other's frame of reference. Although empathy has connotations of understanding the emotional state of another individual, it is unlikely that full understanding is possible, especially with people who have dementia. It is a challenge to imagine the frame of reference in terms of which a person with dementia experiences the world. However, if they dare to look, for most people their own times of abandonment, betrayal, or being outpaced will offer some insight into what a person with dementia is going through. The more a caregiver knows about the "normal" life events and places from the resident's past, the more he or she can relate to the resident as somebody who is "knowable." One staff member mentioned:

This makes you feel that the residents are real people. As I know about Pauline's homes and other things from her past, I can see how difficult it must have been for her and her family.

Getting to know the past can help create empathetic identification that transcends the "job" aspect of caregiving and can help the staff cope with the demanding and emotionally exhausting nature of dementia care. Several responses indicated that getting to know the earlier history of the residents could help the staff approach the daily routine of work on a more humane level. The nurse manager of a nursing home commented:

> *You try to do your job. But sometimes it's really hard . . . to not forget that these are people with history, who had their own lives, like normal people. I want to know them, to feel them, as regular folks. If they can't speak for themselves, somebody else needs to. The biosketches made me look at them as people I know, and this helps me interact with them with feeling—not just doing it as a job.*

A number of staff members commented that knowledge of the person's homes and home-related personal life stories acted as a buffer against job-related stress and in some instances helped them find their jobs more meaningful. Although the primary purpose of home stories is to provide a resource or a tool for use in planning care and activities for persons with dementia, the process can contribute positively to staff members' perceptions of their jobs. This assessment is captured in this comment:

> *I feel that I can help those residents better. I know them like I know my mother or aunt, and somehow, this knowing has helped me connect with them better—both technically, jobwise, and emotionally. I wish I had place-biosketches for all the residents here. That will give a new meaning to my work.*

Developing and Using Home Stories

If the benefits of home stories are to be realized in day-to-day care for persons with dementia, caregivers and staff members need practical guidance on how to develop and use these tools. The staff members at a typical care facility are overworked, and any additional task may seem daunting. A key factor, then, is organizational commitment to encouraging and supporting collaboration among staff, family and friends, and volunteers to develop home stories as resources in dementia care.

From the facility's perspective, any staff member or volunteer can take the initiative to begin a home story project. Families and friends play a critical role and need to be informed about the value and objective of home stories. Although family members may intuitively appreciate the utility of such a biographical approach, they are unlikely to grasp its full potential. Volunteers may be a valuable resource in providing leadership for the project and may be asked to coordinate the activities involved in collecting information from families.

The primary purpose of home stories is to inform caregivers and staff members about residents' history and to enable caregivers to use that information as verbal and visual prompts in guided conversation sessions. As I noted earlier, personal photographs of past homes and specific questions about events associated with homes and other places are generally much more powerful in eliciting a response than a generic photograph or general question. Home stories should be read by all the staff, not just by the activity staff. The nursing staff, including care aides, interact the most with residents, and while they may not be participating in any organized conversation or activity, they can bring up the topic of home as they are interacting with a resident in daily activities. Activity staff members have the opportunity to use the information in the planned activities and conversation sessions with small groups of residents.

In their responses to the home stories I shared and in focus group conversations, the staff members I worked with suggested that the following questions are helpful in eliciting key life-story information related to home and other meaningful places. (Obviously, there could be other questions more relevant to individual circumstances.)

HOMES AND PLACES IN CHILDHOOD YEARS

- Where did your loved one live during childhood (cities, neighborhoods, villages)?
- Can you describe that neighborhood?
- Do you know about the home(s) your loved one lived in during childhood?
- Can you describe those homes?
- Did your loved one have a favorite room or space?
- Was any home and/or neighborhood special to your loved one? If so, what was special about that place?

- Did your loved one travel to any place as a child?
- Did your loved one talk about homes or any other place from her or his childhood?

HOMES AND PLACES IN ADULT YEARS

- Where did your loved one live during adulthood (cities, neighborhoods, villages)?
- Can you describe the physical and social characteristics of the houses/housing (e.g., single-family home, apartment)?
- Are there homes that might be especially meaningful to your loved one? If so, why?
- Was there any home that she or he did not like for some reason? If so, why?
- Was there any space/area in a home that your loved one particularly liked/valued? If so, why?
- What were the things your loved one used to do at home (e.g., cooking, cleaning, redecorating)?
- Did your loved one have any interest in gardens or gardening? If so, what were the activities she or he used to do in gardens or yards?
- What emotions might your loved one have about any of her or his past home(s)?
- Can you describe physical and social characteristics of the neighborhoods of your loved one's homes (e.g., suburb/central city, neighborliness, community activities)?
- What were the places that she or he had traveled to outside the city?
- Was there any place that she or he wanted to go, but could not or did not?
- Where was your loved one living before moving into the care facility?
- If your loved one moved here from another facility, where was her or his last residence in a community?

Photographs and Other Artifacts

Pictures are powerful triggers of recollection. Home stories tend to be more effective when they include visual materials. Photographs are channels that allow us to communicate with the person who has difficulty understanding word-based communications, and personal family photographs provide an excellent visual link to the reality of the person with dementia. In addition to photographs, there may be other objects from the past that the person might relate to. Family members could be asked to identify a few objects in the person's home (including even items of furniture) that he or she has a special memory of.

Small Groups Can Work

Reminiscence sessions with two to four individuals who have dementia may sometimes work positively, depending on the personal dynamics among the residents and the skills of the activity staff member offering the session. When a group works well, one resident's recollection may enable another to recall or connect to her or his past and to communicate that memory. So there is a potential for positive synergy in a small group in which the individuals want to participate and are able to connect with the topic at hand. However, it is critical that the staff member leading the group be familiar with all the residents in the group, have developed relationships with them before the session, and be able to moderate the session in a compassionate and understanding manner.

Consider the Location

Reminiscence sessions should take place where the person with dementia is comfortable. It may be the resident's room, a quiet lounge, or a quiet area in the garden. It is important to reduce distractions and unnecessary stimulation. Often, the social spaces in care facilities (the dining and activity areas) have high levels of stimulation from the noise, activities, movements, and presence of other residents. A place of reminiscence should be calming and helpful in focusing the resident's attention to the topic of home. However, depending on the circumstances, reminiscence sessions can be started with a seated group of residents in the dining space or the main activity space. The primary concern is to regulate distractions that may arise because of staff movement, television, or other sensory stimuli that compete for attention.

The Time of Day

Different times of day work differently for different individuals. However, in general, persons with dementia may be more restless in the late afternoon because of staff shift changes, reduced daylight ("sundowning"), and other factors. Late morning is generally a time when people with dementia are less restless and better able to focus and cooperate. Identify the time of day when a person may be less restless and more cooperative, and be flexible in offering reminiscence sessions based on the individual's schedule. The last thing a staff member should do is impose a session on the resident, because doing so can make the person agitated or aggressive.

Connect and Affirm the Reality of the Person with Dementia

Do not contradict or correct the person when she or he might be relating something "inaccurate," such as "I am going home to finish my work this afternoon." Any reference to home or place can be an opportunity to talk about home in a positive way. Try to affirm the resident's intention about going home and then say something like, "Do you want to talk about what you like about your home?" One must be careful with residents who become easily agitated or upset when they start talking about home. Remembering and talking about home is not an activity that will work for everyone. But if there is an opportunity to have a conversation session with a resident or a small group of residents on home-related experiences, it is critical to accept their recollections as their truth and work with that reality.

Pay attention to nonverbal expressions. Even a resident who is not verbally participating may smile or laugh. This may be an expression based on a feeling connected to the discussion or simply an instinctive response to the social situation. Affirming that feeling is a positive reinforcement for that person. On the other hand, a resident may feel uncomfortable and express anxiety through facial expressions. Those too need to be acknowledged, and the staff member can direct her or his attention to that resident to comfort the person and, if need be, change the focus of the session.

The Length of the Session

Conversation sessions must be flexible as to length. Anyone who conducts activity sessions with persons who have dementia is aware that although structure is important, there must be built-in flexibility as to how the individuals might participate and the length of the session. It is best to think of conversation sessions in terms of short periods of time: 15–20 minutes. Some residents may want to talk or be with the group for longer periods of time, while others may become restless after just a few minutes. Moreover, if reminiscence sessions are thought of as informal and are planned for only short periods, staff members are less likely to become frustrated if the activity cannot be sustained for long.

Family as an Ally

Family members are key resources for developing residents' home stories. As mentioned earlier, ideally the creation of home stories is a collaborative project between staff/volunteers and families. In such a scenario, family members take active responsibility for providing the information sought and may take the initiative to develop a home story, that is, to write the story, incorporate photographs, and so on. Interested family members may volunteer to contact other individuals in the family or friends who are currently not directly involved with the resident's affairs but have relevant biographical information. These may include the resident's childhood friends, siblings, classmates, or colleagues from the workplace. If such individuals live in a different city, they might be contacted by phone or mail and, if they are willing, could be sent a set of questions to respond to.

Beyond helping with or taking the initiative in developing their loved one's home stories, some family members may be interested in conducting guided conversation sessions. It is not uncommon for family members who visit regularly to know other residents beyond their loved ones. If home stories of those residents are available, a family member may want to learn more about those residents' homes and to conduct sessions with them along with her or his own loved one.

Shared Interests and Compatible Dispositions

When planning guided conversation group sessions, it is helpful to select residents who have somewhat similar home experiences. For example, residents who grew up on farms are likely to have common memories of home that can trigger recollection; those who had siblings might have participated in similar activities in the home and neighborhood; those who grew up in the early part of the twentieth century might have attended one-room schoolhouses; and so on.

Although common residential and place experiences may help connect residents with each other, the disposition or personality of the residents is equally relevant when selecting participants for a group activity. Staff members are usually aware of the personality types of the residents. Typically, some residents are more socially interactive than others, some are more restless, and some hardly talk. There is no easy rule to follow. Some individuals get along best with people of their own personality type, while others get along best with people different from themselves. The point is not to suggest any particular combination but to raise the issue as something to consider when inviting and grouping residents for a session.

Closing a Session/Conversation

Any session or conversation related to home or other places from the past must be brought to a close gracefully. The resident who is remembering home needs to feel a sense of achievement and, one hopes, a sense of positive mood. The staff member may close a conversation with a statement such as, "You have a good home and a good life" or "We will talk about your home again." A resident who becomes emotional when talking about her home should not be left alone with no one to listen to or comfort her. It is not uncommon for a resident to become emotional when remembering home, and in that situation the person needs comfort and support (shown through both physical touch and comforting words); in such circumstances, a graceful closure becomes especially important.

Staff Team-Building

Home stories can be used among staff members on a regular basis for reconnecting to the person behind the "resident." This can take different forms, depending on staff preference or routine. One example of such activities is a five-minute home story read-aloud session during lunch that will give information about one resident's homes and places to whichever staff members are present. Visual home stories can be developed and presented as a slide show at the end of care-planning meetings. Attractive displays of photographs and key information can be posted in common spaces in the unit. These activities among the staff members can provide a positive distraction from the typical routine of task-oriented discussions and can help deinstitutionalize the culture of dementia care.

Home Stories as Part of the Culture of Dementia Care

Whether they are used to guide reminiscence sessions with residents, engage family members and volunteers in enhancing the quality of care, or build cohesiveness among caregivers, home stories have one primary goal: to recognize, promote, and support the personhood of individuals with dementia. Learning as much as possible about a person's place-related life experiences from family, friends, former co-workers, and others who knew the individual at various points in his or her life helps caregivers and other staff members come to know the person as a full human being with rich life experiences. For the most part, caregivers do not have access to information about residents' past homes, neighborhoods, farms, villages, and cities that would let them see beyond the condition of dementia and try to connect in ways that are personally meaningful to the individual. Although social workers or staff members in many care facilities develop life stories, those life stories often remain broad and fairly limited. This book makes the case for a focused life story, a home story that is based on the history of homes and places unique to the individual. Home stories, I have argued, are resources that can help caregivers to better understand the resident as a *person* and enable the staff to engage residents in conversations around personally relevant prompts that could connect with the remaining memory of the individual.

This approach is grounded in the larger understanding that the self or the person is always there, no matter what the external conditions may be. It is *our* inability to connect with the person, not just the condition of dementia, that disrupts or breaks down communication. We must remind ourselves, time and again, that the spirit of the person is here as truly as we are here. We must understand and work with the condition of dementia without compromising the human condition of those whom it affects.

Boschetti, M. A. 1984. *The older person's emotional attachment to the physical environment of the residential setting.* Doctoral dissertation, University of Michigan.

Bradford Dementia Groups. 1997. *Evaluating Dementia Care: The DCM Method* (7th ed.). Bradford, UK: University of Bradford.

Brawley, E. 2005. *Design Innovations for Aging and Alzheimer's: Creating Caring Environments.* Wiley: New York.

Brooker, D., & Duce, L. 2000. *Aging and Mental Health 4* (4), 354–58.

Burnham, R. 1998. *Housing Ourselves.* New York: McGraw-Hill.

Butler, R. N. 1963. The life review: An interpretation of reminiscence in the aged. *Psychiatry 26,* 65–76.

Chaudhury, H. 2003. Quality of life and place-therapy. *Journal of Housing for the Elderly* 17(1/2), 85–103.

Cohen, U., & Weisman, G. 1991. *Holding On to Home.* Baltimore: Johns Hopkins University Press.

Csikszentmihalyi, M. 1993. *The Evolving Self: A Psychology for the Third Millennium.* New York: HarperPerennial.

Csikszentmihalyi, M., & Rochberg-Halton, E. 1981. *The Meaning of Things: Domestic Symbols and the Self.* Cambridge: Cambridge University Press.

DeBaggio, T. 2002. *Losing My Mind: An Intimate Look at Life with Alzheimer's.* New York: Free Press.

DeBaggio, T. 2003. *When It Gets Dark: An Enlightened Reflection on Life with Alzheimer's.* New York: Free Press.

Gibson, F. 1994. What can reminiscence contribute to people with dementia. In J. Bornat (Ed.), *Reminiscence Reviewed: Evaluations, Achievements, Perspectives.* Buckingham: Open University Press.

Gibson, F. 2004. *The Past in the Present: Using Reminiscence in Health and Social Care.* Baltimore: Health Professions Press.

Gotell, E., Brown, S., & Ekman, S. 2002. Caregiver singing and background music in dementia care. *Western Journal of Nursing Research* 24(2), 195–216.

Gubrium, J. F. 1993. *Speaking of Life: Horizons of Meaning for Nursing Home Residents.* New York: Aldine de Gruyter.

Haight, B. K. 1991. Reminiscing: The state of the art as a basis for practice. *International Journal of Aging and Human Development 33*, 1–32.

Hall, E. 1969. *The Hidden Dimension.* New York: Doubleday.

Harris, P. B. (Ed.). 2002. *The Person with Alzheimer's Disease: Pathways to Understanding the Experience.* Baltimore: Johns Hopkins University Press.

Henderson, C. 1998. *Partial View: An Alzheimer's Journal.* Dallas: Southern Methodist University Press.

Henderson, J. N. 1995. The culture of care in a nursing home: Effects of a medicalized model of long term care. In J. N. Henderson & M. D. Vesperi (Eds.), *The Culture of Long Term Care: Nursing Home Ethnography.* London: Bergin & Garvey.

Hughes, J. C., Louw, S. J., & Sabat, S. R. 2006. Seeing whole. In J. C. Hughes, S. J. Louw, & S. R. Sabat (Eds.), *Dementia: Mind, Meaning and the Person.* New York: Oxford University Press.

James, W. 1890. *The Principles of Psychology.* Cambridge, New York: Holt.

Jung, C. G. 1989. *Memories, Dreams, Reflections.* New York: Vintage Books.

Kane, M. N. 2003. Teaching direct practice for work with elders with Alzheimer's disease: A simulated group experience. *Education Gerontology 29*(9), 777–94.

Kitwood, T. 1997. *Dementia Reconsidered: The Person Comes First.* Buckingham: Open University Press.

Kitwood, T., & Bredin, K. 1992. Towards a theory of dementia care: Personhood and well-being. *Ageing and Society 12*(3), 269–87.

Kovach, C. R., & Henschel, H. 1996. Planning activities for patients with dementia: A descriptive study of therapeutic activities on special care units. *Journal of Gerontological Nursing 22*(9), 33–38.

Lawton, M. P. 1983. Environments and other determinants of well-being in older people. *Gerontologist 23*, 34–7.

Lieberman, M. A., & Tobin, S. S. 1983. *The Experience of Old Age: Stress, Coping and Survival.* New York: Basic Books.

Marcus, C. C. 1977. *Houses as a Mirror of Self: Exploring the Deeper Meaning of Home.* Newburyport, MA: Conari Press.

Moos, I., & Bjorn, A. 2006. Use of the life story in the institutional care of people with dementia: A review of intervention studies. *Ageing and Society 26*, 431–54.

Moos, R. H., & Lemke, S. 1994. *Group Residences for Older Adults: Physical Features, Policies, and Social Climate.* New York: Oxford University Press.

Moss, S. E., Polignano, E., White, C. L., Minichiello, M. D., & Sunderland, T. 2002. Reminiscence group activities and discourse interaction in Alzheimers disease. *Journal of Gerontological Nursing 28*(8), 36–44.

Neisser, U. 1994. Self-narratives: True or false. In U. Neisser & R. Fivush (Eds.), *The Remembering Self.* Cambridge: Cambridge University Press.

Patton, M. Q. 2002. *Qualitative Research and Evaluation Methods*. Newbury Park, CA: Sage.

Piper, A. I., & Langer, E. J. 1986. Aging and mindful control. In M. M. Baltes & P. B. Baltes (Eds.), *The Psychology of Control and Aging*. Hillsdale, NJ: Erlbaum.

Polkinghorne, D. E. 1988. *Narrative Knowing and the Human Sciences*. New York: SUNY Press.

Proshansky, H. M., Fabian, A. K., & Kaminoff, R. 1983. Place identity: Physical world socialization of the self. *Journal of Environmental Psychology 3*, 57–83.

Ricoeur, P. 1992. *Oneself as Another* (K. Blamey, Trans.). Chicago: University of Chicago Press.

Rowles, G. D. 1978. *Prisoners of Space? Exploring the Geographical Experience of Older People*. Boulder, CO: Westview Press.

Rowles, G. D. 1980. Toward a geography of growing old. In A. Buttimer & D. Seamon (Eds.), *The Human Experience of Space and Place*. London: Croom Helm.

Rowles, G. D. 1983. Place and personal identity in old age: Observations from Appalachia. *Journal of Environmental Psychology 3*, 299–313.

Rowles, G. D. 1993. Evolving images of place in aging and aging in place. *Generations 17*(2), 65–70.

Rowles, G., & Chaudhury, H. (Eds.). 2005. *Home and Identity in Late Life: International Perspectives*. New York: Springer.

Rubinstein, R. L. 1989. The home environments of older people: A description of psychological processes linking person to place. *Journal of Gerontology 44*, S44–S53.

Rubinstein, R. L., & Parmelee, P. A. 1992. Attachment to place and the representation of the life course by the elderly. In I. Altman & S. M. Low (Eds.), *Place Attachment*. New York: Plenum.

Sabat, S. R. 2001. *The Experience of Alzheimer's Disease: Life through a Tangled Veil*. Oxford: Blackwell.

Sabat, S. R. 2002. Surviving manifestations of selfhood in Alzheimer's disease: A case study. *Dementia 1*(1), 25–36.

Sherman, E. 1995. Reminiscentia: Cherished objects as memorabilia in late-life reminiscence. In J. Hendricks (Ed.), *The Meaning of Reminiscence and Life Review*. Amityville, NY: Baywood.

Stokols, D., & Shumaker, S. A. 1981. People in places: A transactional view of settings. In J. H. Harvey (Ed.), *Cognition, Social Behavior, and the Environment*. Hillsdale, NJ: Erlbaum.

Tan, A. 1995. *Rules of the Game*. New York: Ivy Books.

Thorgrimsen, L., Schweitzer, P., & Orrell, M. 2002. Evaluating reminiscence for people with dementia: A pilot study. *The Arts in Psychotherapy 29*, 93–97.

Weisman, G. D., Chaudhury, H., & Moore, K. D. 2000. Theory and practice of place: Toward an integrative model. In R. Rubinstein, M. Moss, & M. H. Kleban (Eds.), *The Many Dimensions of Aging*. New York: Springer.

White, E. B. 1952. *Charlotte's Web*. New York: Harper & Row.

Woods, R. T., & McKiernan, F. 1995. Evaluating the impact of reminiscence on older people with dementia. In B. K. Haight & J. D. Webster (Eds.), *The Art and Science of Reminiscing: Theory, Research, Methods, and Applications*. Washington, DC: Taylor & Francis.

About the Author

Habib Chaudhury is assistant professor in the Department of Gerontology at Simon Fraser University, in Vancouver, British Columbia, Canada. He is also affiliated with the Centre for Research on Personhood in Dementia at the University of British Columbia. He holds a Ph.D. in architecture / environment-behavior studies from the University of Wisconsin–Milwaukee. His research interests include aging and environment, place-therapy for persons with dementia, self and dementia, design for people with dementia, design for active living, and design of health care environments. He is the co-editor (with Graham Rowles) of *Home and Identity in Late Life*.